Physical therapists across the country with several hundred combined years of physical therapy practice were asked to provide their own self-created solutions to 100 very commonly occurring but challenging clinical scenarios that their PT school program could have never prepared them for. Although these scenarios are very common, each occurrence is always specific to the circumstance and individually unique, so the answers/solutions to these scenarios cannot be cited in text books or taught in a classroom. However, through their many years of clinical practice and experience, individual physical therapists have created and utilized hundreds of effective practical solutions to these challenging clinical scenarios to improve their own clinical practice. Unfortunately, new physical therapists typically must practice for many years in order gain enough experience to develop their own solutions to these clinical scenarios. The goal of collecting these physical therapist-created clinical practical solutions was to make them available to new physical therapists to use as modifiable templates as they formulate their own individual solutions to the same common challenging scenarios, but without waiting years to gain enough experience to do it alone.

Contents

7

8

How do I respectfully tell a patient to leave their family/friends in the waiting room or not bring them at all?

There are times when a patient has children who are disruptive and can even be a safety concern in a physical therapy gym. Patient may not want others such as friends, parents, and other relatives to hear sensitive information, and thus not give important and valuable information during evaluations and follow ups. However, the other party may feel that it is their right to stay with their loved one, and take offense to you asking them not to stay with the patient. You can lose valuable respect from your patient if you go about this in the wrong way, and if you seem rude and cold, you may ruin an opportunity to make a positive impression on the patient's loved one who is often a potential patient in the future. The following are some ideas from other veteran physical therapists.

- Prior to the initiation of the evaluation, I request that family members are only present if they can aide in answering questions for patient. (Ex: pt is unable to communicate or has aphasia).

- Explain to the family/friends that you need to respect the patient's privacy by speaking to them alone. Then invite them to hang out in the waiting room, and have some coffee. Tell them that you will be happy to answer any of their questions or concerns after you have completed your evaluation of the patient.

- If there is a nurse involved, as in a hospital setting, ask the nurse to have the family wait in the waiting room before you go in the room.

- Allow the family to ask one question. Only answer that one question, and then say "if you have any more questions at the end I will be happy to answer them. In the meantime, can I have you guys wait in the waiting room while I focus on the patient? Thanks". Then physically turn your body toward the patient and continue with the evaluation.

- Let them know that you are interested in what they have to say, but that you would need some quiet time with the patient

11

to do a full evaluation and then you would be happy to talk with them after the evaluation is complete.

- "I am committed to getting your mom well with to my best abilities. In order for me to do a good job, I will need your cooperation by staying in the waiting room, so I can best help your mom".

- Tell them that I understand their concerns and will be happy discuss them after I have completed my evaluation.

"Prior to the evaluation, I ask that only the family/friends who can answer important questions remain in the room". Jaisie Stevens. DPT. Washington, DC

- Use language that strongly suggests that you only want the patient in the treatment room, and be stern about it, but don't make it a big deal. Say things like: "give us a few minutes, this won't take too long, ok".

- "when we are done with the initial evaluation, I'll come and get you and you can ask me any questions you may have".

- "are you with Mr. Smith? Ok, please wait here until we are done".

- "Excuse me, I need equipment in another area to complete this evaluation, we will be back shortly".

- Use the phrase "Allow me to work with Mr. Smith one-on-one" This avoids the possibility of insulting the patients loved one, and puts them at ease if they are an adult by essentially asking permission to treat their loved one without them being present.

- If the problem is disruptive children, and if there is another guardian around, first simply smile and say "better leave the kids here until we are done". Later, when you have a chance, apologize and explain to the patient that the kids may be a "little bit" disruptive, and that you need to direct all of your attention to them and their physical problem in order to fix it. This may allow the patient to see that you are really attempting to do your best to help them, and allows them to assist in that process.

- If the problem is children being a safety concern in the PT gym, simply explain that although there are a lot of fun things all around for the kids to play with, and since you (the patient) will be very busy with therapy and won't be able to closely watch them, it really can become a dangerous situation for their child/children.

- Most parents will probably understand, especially considering the safety of their children, and won't bring them to the next session with them if at all possible.

- If it is a cognizant adult, I would ask to see the patient privately for a moment and ask them if they are comfortable with the interruptions. If they are then I would try to incorporate the family into the session and make them a team player. If the patient it is not comfortable I would ask to see the family member alone and share the patient's concerns. If it is a kiddo, I probably would ask the parent what their major concerns are and ask if we could discuss them at the end of the session instead of no

How would I explain in layman's terms how ultrasound works?

No one likes a smartass who acts like he knows it all, even if he/she is the physical therapist. No one likes to listen to what sounds like babble in foreign language either. And no one likes a health practioner who treats them in a condescending manner as if they are not smart enough to understand what is being said to them. Remember that people tend to expect machines to make noises, flash lights or make motions in order to be effective, and ultrasound does not necessarily do any of these. So, don't be too surprised if a patient thinks that it's just smoke and mirrors, and that an ultrasound head is just some type of massage tool that's used to spread massage lotion around on a person's skin. If they ask what it does, it may mean that they feel somewhat uneasy about having this procedure performed on them, and they want to make sure that they are getting quality and legitimate treatment. It would not be wise to miss this opportunity to gain more respect from your patient while educating them and putting their mind at ease. However, even though you know very well how ultrasound works, if you sound as if you are not sure, the patient's suspicions will only worsen. Here are some suggestions.

- Describe ultrasound as a therapeutic procedure which uses sound waves to provide an internal micro-massage to the deep tissues to reduce stiffness and to promote healing with (or without) heat and micro-vibrations. The sound waves are above the level of human hearing, and they penetrate into the soft tissue to warm and relax tension, to improve circulation and reduce pain. Depending on the setting, the patient may feel a comfortable warming effect as the transducer is moved around in massaging strokes, but not pain or intense heat. It is a natural physical agent to promote better soft tissue mobility.

- Ultrasound uses variable frequency sound waves to penetrate your tissues and break up scar tissue adhesions that hold your tissues in tight painful positions, allowing more freedom of movement with less pain.

- It emits high-frequency sound waves that cannot be perceived by the human ear. These waves penetrate deeply, causing an increase both in temperature and in blood flow, which leads to faster healing.

- Ultrasound treatment is used to deliver penetrating heat deep within your tissues. Soft tissues are like plastic in that when it's cold it is rigid and difficult to stretch, but when warm, it becomes more pliable and can be stretched easily.

- Ultrasound increases the local circulation within your tissues by increasing the heat deep within. This speeds the healing process.

14

- Unlike diagnostic ultrasound which is used in hospitals to see structures in your body such as a pregnant woman's fetus, this is therapeutic ultrasound, and it uses more powerful ultrasound waves to heat soft tissue and speed healing time by loosening tight soft tissue, increase blood circulation, and breakdown scar tissue.

- Ultrasound delivers direct heat to the area of injury, and it reduces swelling and inflammation which are the main sources of pain. This heating effect also increases blood flow in the treated area which speeds the healing process.

- Ultrasound emits anywhere between one and three million vibrations of sound waves per second to penetrate your soft tissues and loosen painfully tight muscles, tendons, and ligaments.

- With injured tissues, ultrasound speeds the rate of healing and enhance the quality of tissue repair by decreasing inflammation and improving local blood supply to the injured site.

- Ultrasound helps your condition in many ways. It improves the blood supply to the injured area, which helps speed recovery. It causes painfully tight tissues to relax, which decreases your pain. It also breaks up scar tissue so that healing will be more efficient, which reduces the chance of re-injury.

- Ultrasound is used to heat soft tissues that are deeper than can be reached with moist heat. Moist heat only heats to approximately 1-2 centimeters deep, while ultrasound heats 1-5 centimeters deep. The heating effect causes tight tissues such as spastic muscles to relax. It also improves the blood supply, which speeds the healing process so that you can recover faster.

- Ultrasound works on the cellular level and stimulates the injured tissues to repair faster by enhancing the cell-repair effects of the inflammation process.

- Ultrasound uses variable frequency sound waves to penetrate your tissues and break up scar tissue adhesions that hold your tissues in tight painful positions, allowing more freedom of movement with less pain.

- Ultrasound treatment is used to deliver penetrating heat deep within your tissues. Soft tissues are like plastic in that when it's cold it is rigid and difficult to stretch, but when warm, it becomes more pliable and can be stretched easily.

- Ultrasound increases the local circulation within your tissues by increasing the heat deep within. This speeds the healing process.

- Soft tissues such as muscles, ligaments, tendons, joint capsules, and fascia, are basically a collection of thousands upon thousands of cells which reproduces on itself until the tissue is formed. If the tissue is injured the cells begin reproducing again in order to repair the damaged tissue. On this cellular level, ultrasound alters cell membrane permeability, structure, and function, which simulates tissue repair.

How would I briefly explain in layman's terms how electrical stimulation works?

People generally react negatively toward the unknown. That goes double for electrical stimulation. This is because there is a strange machine being attached to their body, which is probably already injured or in pain. And in addition to simply not knowing what it does, the patient feels the electrical current and may become afraid of being "shocked" or hurt in some way. They may even initially refuse the treatment. And if they are a new patient and they know that you are a new therapist, their lack of confidence in your competent use of such a "scary" "dangerous" machine may come to the surface. You as the Physical Therapist are charged with the responsibility of placing the patient's mind at ease so that treatment can be performed effectively. Here are some suggestions:

- Electrical stimulation helps their muscles to contract, thereby helping them to re-learn how to use the muscle more effectively.

- If explaining how it works to decrease pain, I explain to them that it helps to lower pain threshold just like when you bump your arm and rub it. You rub it to make it feel good. What is really happening is, touch sensation and pain sensation go to the same area of the brain. Touch just has a faster car. That way you are telling your brain you don't have pain here. E-stim works the same way just with electrical pulses vs. touching the area.

- I explain the pain signals are like a loud annoying voice you do not want to hear, so you turn on a louder radio to drown out the annoying noise. The electrical current helps to drown out the sharper pain sensation, replacing it with gentle tingling sensations. This is what we call the Gate Control Theory for Pain. The current should feel comfortable and should lower their pain level.

- Explain to the patient that there are many forms of electrical stimulation. As for e-stim for pain control, the feeling from the electricity acts upon the same areas that sense pain thus blocking the pain sensation from registering in the brain.

"Electrical Stimulation helps decrease pain by blocking pain signals to the brain". Brett Rice. MPT, FAAOMPT. New Market, MD

- Explain to them that in an uninjured muscle, the brain sends an electrical signal to the muscle which makes it contract at any given time. However, when injured, the signal is not as strong as it needs to be, and the muscle can't do what it needs to do. It's almost as if the muscle never gets the signal. E-stim is a way to send artificial electrical brain signals to the muscles to make them react until the natural signals start working more efficiently.

- Electrical stimulation is used to decrease pain by blocking the pain signal which comes from the injury site and travels to the brain. You are in too much pain for us to do certain things (like manual therapy or therapeutic exercise). This temporary decrease in pain may be enough to make it possible for us to treat the root cause of the problem.

- Your brain produces natural pain reducing chemicals which act much in the same way as aspirin or Tylenol. Depending on the settings and type of current, electrical stimulation can cause your brain to release these natural pain reducing chemicals. This makes the pain much more tolerable.

- To ease the patient's anxiousness and fear, you can say:
  "It might feel kinda funny at first, but it won't hurt"
  "You will feel a slight tingling sensation, that's all"
  "I will turn it up very slowly until you tell me to stop"
  "Simply tell me to stop just before it gets uncomfortable"

- Electrical stimulation can be used for many things. In your case, we use it to reduce the sensation of pain. Depending on the setting we choose, it works by either "scrambling" pain signals to the brain to mask feelings of pain, or by causing the body to produce natural pain-killers called endorphins.

- After surgery or in cases of stroke or severe injury to a muscle, the muscle loses the ability to contract. Electrical stimulation can be used to cause muscles to tense and teach them to contract again by mimicking the natural signals that your brain sends to the muscle which tell it to contract at will.

- Electrical stimulation decreases pain by two different mechanisms. First, electrical stimulation of the nerve can block a pain signal from being carried to the brain. If the signal is blocked, pain is not perceived. Secondly, it causes the body to release natural chemicals called endorphins which suppress pain. These chemicals are very similar to the active ingredients in pain medication.

- Following surgery or severe trauma to muscles, they sometimes become too weak to contract in the manner that they did prior to injury. They need to be strengthened. However, the severe weakness may be an obstacle to strengthening because the muscles may be too weak to actively exercise. Electrical stimulation can then be used to artificially and passively contract the muscle in order to prepare it for active contraction as it gets stronger.

- Severe injury may sometimes cause excessive swelling, which then increases pain. Your body responds to the excess swelling by pumping a little bit out every time the muscle involved contracts and relaxes. However, when the muscle is in too much pain, or is too weak, electrical stimulation can be used to assist with this method of controlling swelling by passively causing a muscle contraction followed by relaxation repeatedly. This is beneficial to you as a patient because it has the effect of decreasing the painful swelling within the tissues.

- When there is a nerve injury involved, and the "message" from the brain is having difficulty reaching the desired muscle through the normal pathway to cause it to move, electrical stimulation can be used to "reteach" the brain how to do it by sending the message repeatedly until the brain re-learns a different pathway to the muscle.

How would I explain in layman's terms how muscles get stronger?

In general, most people know that your muscles get stronger when you exercise. However, some pts want to know the mechanism behind it. In fact, this question arises very often during the standard PT-pt interaction. If you as the therapist can easily communicate the process effortlessly, you may gain more respect from your patient, thus increasing compliance with home exercise and in-clinic activities. Conversely, if the physical therapist cannot effectively communicate the process to the pt, and even if one knows the process well, the opposite may occur, and this could even eventually lead to other negative behaviors such as no-shows and late-shows and non-compliance, because of lack of confidence in his/her therapist. Explaining the complex relationship between muscle fibers, sarcomeres, and hypertrophy will almost always be too much for the average layman to understand. It may also be TMI (too much info), leading to loss of interest. Here are some suggestions on explaining how muscles get stronger.

- When overloaded with weight, the muscle is temporarily damaged. If this is done repeatedly, the body adapts by adding more muscle tissue so that the damage won't happen again.

- I always tell patients the first change in at a neurological level. With repeated use of muscles, your body just gets more efficient. Rather than recruiting all of the little muscle fibers to perform a given task, the brain learns to use the right muscle fibers and just the right amount of them, which requires less effort and causes less fatigue afterward. Once the brain realizes that its still difficult for the muscle to get the job done, it starts building more muscles to help get the job done more efficiently with less effort.

- Explain to the patient that muscles get stronger when they are challenged beyond their normal activity, so we need to challenge their muscles through specific therapeutic exercise.

- Everyone knows the phrase, " If you don't use it, you lose it." Muscle gains strength by proper use on a regular basis. If the muscles are not active, they respond by reducing their size and ability to produce force. When muscles are challenged, they respond by becoming larger, known as hypertrophy. They may also add more muscle cells or fibers, resulting in what we notice as the larger muscles. Because there are larger muscle cells or even additional muscle cells, the muscle is able to generate more force with less effort, making it easier to lift, push and pull items for everyday function. Therapists are educated to determine the necessary workload required to promote muscle growth and development within a safe training intensity. A workout may be uncomfortable, but it should not be painful. We challenge the muscle by providing just the right amount of resistance, adequate set, repetitions and rest periods to enable the muscle to safely improve its function.

- First your body gets better at using your muscles. When you pick something up, only a portion of the small fibers of muscles are used. As you train your body, it begins to use more and more of the available muscle fibers, which work together to make you stronger. After that, when you work to strengthen a muscle, you cause little tears, or trauma to the muscle fibers which grow bigger as they heal.

- Microscopic damage is made with heavy resistance, and the body takes a little time as it replaces the torn muscle fibers with more and stronger fibers

- Your body senses when a new and recurring demand on muscles is too great, and compensates by adding more muscle fibers to aide in the increased demand.

- Muscles have a need to be strong enough to work efficiently with the least amount of effort as possible every day. When you repeatedly place a demand on the muscle which requires too much effort, the body automatically starts building the muscle up stronger and bigger so that less effort will be needed to handle that demand. But like gaining weight, it takes time.

- Your body is made in a way that it "learns" from experience. When you put more stress on your muscles than you usually do while performing a particular activity, it "remembers" the excess stress, and builds more muscle so that it can easily handle the stress the next time.

- When you have a cut in your skin, your body repairs the cut and overcompensates by leaving a scar. When you rub your hands raw, your body repairs the skin and overcompensates by rebuilding the skin until there are callouses formed. The same is true for your muscles. When you lift heavy weight, you actually cause micro- injury to your muscles. Your body overcompensates for lack of ability to prevent an injury by building up the injured body part greater than it was before the injury.

- Muscle get stronger through the "destroy and rebuild" theory of exercise. Forcing your muscles to move a heavy load injures the muscle on a microscopic level. It "destroys the muscle". Your body "rebuilds" the muscle bigger and stronger than it was before the "destruction". The more this is done, the bigger the muscle becomes.

What's the best way to inform a patient that they have a very foul odor and need to address it?

Apparently, this occurs a lot in outpatient as well as in-patient settings. It may be somewhat easier to address in an in-patient setting because the patient is "living" in the facility, and personal hygiene/grooming may be integrated into the daily concerns of the patient's therapy team which may include nursing, OT, nursing assistants, and others. In this case the patient understands that professionals may be partly responsible with helping him/her with self-care, and may welcome any feedback on hygiene. In an outpatient setting, it may be much more difficult to address this problem because the patient is usually relatively independent with self-care, and may get offended if his/her cleanliness is called into question. You as the therapist do not want to offend your patient, as it may lead to other undesirable consequences such as effecting the patient's enthusiasm, lead to improper performance of exercise, and lack of compliance with scheduled sessions because of embarrassment, not to mention your own extreme embarrassment if he/she took offence to what you tell them. Relax, here are some ideas and suggestions:

- I have had some patients show up for therapy after working on car transmissions in the heat all day. They came to their appointment covered in grease and dirt, sweaty and ripe. It was so bad that other patients remarked they were offended by the odor! I had to ask the patients gracefully to return home to shower, and welcomed them to return later in the day for therapy. It was very clear to them they were offensive, and they laughed and said they did not want to be late for PT. I told them I appreciate their courtesy, but I would be better able to serve them without all that dirty grease.

- If the patient is not homeless or is able to afford for laundry facilities, soap, etc., and is capable of taking care of their own hygiene needs, it could be a good opportunity for a chat about how we can best take care of ourselves. In order to avoid embarrassing the patient, frame it as one of the ways we can keep ourselves healthy.

- Inform the patient that there is a difference between good and bad pain, and that you will help them to discern the difference.

- When I worked in the hospitals, some patients were incontinent, presenting a foul odor, or just had problems with excessive perspiration. In that case, I tried to schedule their next visit with the nurses to be seen after their bath.

- In an inpatient setting, I do not complain to patients about a foul odor if it appears they are unable to manage it on their own.

- Vicks vapor rub under the nose is a good short-term solution.

- I offer a patient gown to wear if their clothing is soiled, so it smells fresher.

- For people with very foul-smelling feet, we use a chlorinated whirlpool bath prior to treatment. I have also used rubbing alcohol on a terry towel to freshen patients' feet before treating them.

- The most important thing to remember in this situation is talk to the person in a private area where there are no other patients or PT staff.

- Make sure the patient understands that you are addressing the problem because it is your job to do so, and not merely because you don't like the way they smell.

"Frame the conversation as one of the ways we can keep ourselves healthy". Irene Drizi. PT. Athens, Greece.

- Make the patient aware that you are also addressing the problem because you care for all of your patients, and are concerned about anything that affects them negatively.

- Use your professional expertise on the subject. Address it from a healthcare standpoint by going into the reasons for the smell. Address the fact that some people have sweat glands that produce more sweat than others, and so they need to work harder than the average person to get the same result of washing it from the skin. The key here is to tell them that you can smell them.

- If they are a smoker, you can address it from that angle by explaining the obvious health risks first, and then explaining how cigarette smoking filters toxins into the bloodstream which eventually are secreted through the skin and smells bad. Tell them in a nice way that you can actually smell them and can tell they are a smoker. Be completely honest when telling them that if they don't stop smoking, they will have to wash their skin twice as thorough in order to simply smell clean.

- If the patient simply smells of underarm odor, first do a little research to find a list of hypoallergenic deodorants or antiperspirants for persons with hyper-sensitivity to the chemicals in deodorants. Talk to the patient in private and if it helps, tell them that you have been approached by another person who has the condition, who noticed the smell, and who thought the patient could use the list. The bad part about this method is that there is a small white lie involved. The good part about this suggestion is that it gets the job done without the need to tell the patient that bathing may solve the problem because it gives the patient an option to escape an embarrassing moment by thinking that they are letting you believe the smell is due to a medical problem, and the solution to the problem is to use one of the deodorants on the list. They can then go home, bathe properly, and return for the next session feeling and smelling clean as a whistle. They will expect you to think that the change was due to simply changing the type of deodorant. They will probably attempt to drive that idea home by thanking you for giving them the list. You should then be very gracious in accepting the gratitude, but never bring it up again unless the patient does first, and even then, only discuss it from a physical therapists point of view as it relates to the patient's general health and wellness.

What's a good way to tell a patient that pain and discomfort may be necessary for improvement?

Patients come to physical therapy to alleviate their musculoskeletal problem, and pain is usually a part of their problem. Although it is true in certain situations, most people have a pre-conceived idea that physical therapy is very hard to undergo, and that it is worth the difficulty in the end, the last thing that they want is to be forced to endure is more pain. Patients often miss appointments or are extremely reluctant to fully participate in therapy during their sessions when they are anxious and concerned about the possibility of more pain. This will obviously make your job as the therapist much more difficult, and possibly negatively affect your outcome/results of your treatment. It would be wise of you as the physical therapist to address this problem by putting the patient's mind at ease so that they can come to terms with what must be done. This will make your job much easier and help you achieve better outcome from therapy, which will make you a better physical therapist. Here are some suggestions on how to address this problem.

- I ask patients if they are familiar with the typical "no pain, no gain" statement used by some athletes. I do not agree that pain is a necessary component of improving one's physical condition.

- Tell the patient that pain does not always equal harm, and that they are safe in your hands because you will not allow their pain to reach the level of harm.

- Sometimes, the patient's concern comes from wondering if the pain is signaling that something you are doing is wrong and will hurt them in the long run. If this is the case, reassuring them that the type of pain or discomfort they are experiencing is normal will satisfy their concern. In this case, inform the patient that it is common to feel some discomfort with the interventions you are implementing, but to hang on because it does get better.

- A reference to the ancient Greek quote by Epimarchos: "All the good things are gained laboriously", is very useful.

- I tell patients that the body heals through a low grade inflammatory response. If it is just a 1-2/10 and is tolerable they will probably get more out of pushing through that vs. avoiding the movement.

- I acknowledge that when there is injury or disease, pain may be a component of the process related to healing and to tissue damage.

- Tell the patient that the pain calls our attention to the problem to allow us to remove ourselves from the pain-producing issue, or to attend to the physical needs of the body.

- I inform the patient that we must pay attention to the pain, but if it interferes with our daily function, action must be taken to resolve the problem.

- Tell them that when joints and muscles are stiff after an injury, such as when a cast is removed, it will be painful to move initially, but the body must get used to moving again after it has undergone immobilization. Tissues and fascia has shortened with lack of use, and only use and motion will promote lengthening of the tissue.

- Begin with a thorough explanation of their diagnosis and plan of treatment in simple everyday language, and carefully outline what they are to expect, including how long you expect the pain should take to go away. This gives them a "heads up", and allows them to know what to expect instead of being caught off guard by more discomfort. It is very effective in easing the patient's mind about the possibility of experiencing more discomfort during physical therapy, especially if they understand the process by which their symptoms may be relieved. Patients are usually more willing to endure the temporary discomfort if they know how long it should last, why it is present, and that they will feel a lot better after it's over with.

- Use the phrase "it's going to feel worse before it feels better, but when the worst part is over, it's going to feel so much better that it was worth going through the bad part.

26

- Ask the patient for permission to be frank with them. When granted, frankly explain to the patient that he/she could either avoid addressing the problem and deal with the pain without an end in sight, or address the problem head-on and tolerate a little more discomfort for a brief period of time followed by no pain.

- Tell them this story (and it's a true one). I once had a tooth which was infected at the nerve root. I needed a root canal. I put off going to the dentist for a week because I hated the idea of having a dentist drill going into the already painful area. I experienced pain during that week that almost made me lose consciousness at times. I finally made the brave decision to get it over with and have the root canal performed. The procedure was not fun at all, but I remember watching a sitcom on television later the same day I had the root canal, and I remember chuckling about some joke that was not even very funny. The interesting thing is I heard myself laugh. I would not have laughed before the root canal, but the lack of pain allowed me to concentrate on what I was doing, in this case, it was paying attention to the jokes in a sitcom. Suddenly, I realized that the pain was really gone. It's like the sun just came out after a rainy day. And the clouds were brushed aside. Moral of the story: It's better to get it over with than to prolong the agony and live in uncertainty.

- "You may feel mild discomfort after today's session because we did exercises that your body is not used to doing. But it should be very mild and shouldn't last more than a couple days"

- "You can expect some mild muscle soreness within the next 48 hours. It's the "good kind" of soreness, and is very normal. It's just like when you start a new exercise regimen at the gym. For the first few days, you experience a lot of muscle soreness because your muscles are rebuilding".

- "Because you have not been able to move properly for so long, your body has stiffened into that position. It may feel a little worse before it feels better because we have to move your body in ways it has not moved in a while in order loosen it up and get rid of that painful stiffness".

- If the painful condition being treated was not due to trauma, but was instead due to a chronic cause, I explain to the patient that the pain did not come to this point over night, so it won't heal overnight. I then tell them that discomfort during this healing period is expected, but should be temporary and if they can make it through the pain, it will be worth the effort.

- It starts at the initial evaluation. After you have performed all of your tests and measures, and have developed a PT diagnosis and plan of care. Be completely honest with the patient and tell them the "good new" as well as the "bad news". If you expect an arduous and slow recovery, tell them so. Make them understand that it won't be a "bed of roses", but will be well worth it in the end. Try to explain the level of commitment and patience that will be necessary to progress through PT in a way that will invigorate and challenge them, keeping in mind that at some point along the way they will probably lose courage and question whether or not you are helping them, and you will have to reassure them by reiterating the same words again.

- If all else fails, and the patient wants to quit before the pain has resolved, I sometimes implement the "no pain-no gain" theory, and hold no punches when I tell them that if they don't deal with this now, it won't end, and they will be dealing with it for a long time to come.

How do I deal with a situation where a patient is appropriate for discharge, but exaggerate their symptoms in order to stay because they have become emotionally attached to therapy?

We as physical therapists spend much more time caring for our patients than almost any other health care professional. It must be fully understood that human interaction always eventually correlates with human emotion. The more time a person (who happens to be a physical therapist) spends caring for another person (who happens to be a patient), the more emotionally attached that person/patient becomes. Obviously, this is especially true for some patients more than others. Often, you will find a patient exaggerating their symptoms in order to continue physical therapy. Although being nice and feeding into this may initially seem like the right thing to do, it is not. It would be unwise to encourage this because it will seem as if your treatment outcome is not effective. It is also unethical to charge a patient for treatment that is unnecessary. Other reasons are that it makes more work for you as the therapist because you are receiving new patients, but your old patients are still in therapy, so your patient load keeps growing (and we don't need to go into how that can mushroom out of control), also the referring doctor will want to know why his/her patient has not made a full recovery by this time, and many more reasons. Here are some ways to handle this situation:

- Use functional outcome measures at the beginning, and then use it at re-evaluation. If no significant improvement, point to the results as the reason for discharge.

- As qualified physical therapist, we are able to discern what is real and what is not real. It is always important to use objective measurements so that you can manage progression toward your goals. You should keep the patient involved in that progression and if there's nothing more that you can do for the patient, let them know that. It's OK if you maximize their potential. It's OK to tell them that. Put them on a home exercise and discharge them.

- Tell them that there is no more therapeutic benefit that can be achieved by PT.

- If in skilled setting: lets devise a restorative program to maintain your improvements, our restorative aid will be walking with you daily and bringing you to the therapy gym to perform exercises to keep you strong. If returning home, home health PT will come to help transition you to your home, here is your home exercise program, the home health PT may add to it or devise a new one based on her/his assessment within your home.

- Tell the patient that you need to be able to document weekly improvements either on a VAS or with objective finding to differentiate between restorative PT and maintenance PT, because health insurance doesn't cover maintenance PT, and they will be charged out of pocket for maintenance PT.

" Its ok to inform the patient that they have maximized their potential". Cynthia Bell. DPT. Valdosta GA

- Set goals at the beginning and make sure they understand that once the goals have been met, they will be discharged because they no longer need PT. The goals must be measurable and objective, not subjective. When the goals have been met, remind them that it means it is time for discharge.

- If the patient was referred to you by his/her doctor, the patient knows that the doctor is already aware of their status prior to the start of therapy. Make the patient aware that you will be sending documentation about their progress to the doctor. The patient should immediately stop exaggerating because if they are smart, they will realize that the doctor will compare notes and see that they are exaggerating, and that means that their follow-up visit to their doctor will be very embarrassing and uncomfortable.

- I will usually ween them off PT. Start by lowering to 1x/wk, then 1x/every other week. Then I will tell them to try their program on their own for about a month or so. If the problem hasn't gotten better after that month, then come back in. They will usually fall out of the routine by then and be okay.

- Avoid this problem by preparing them for discharge well in advance of the date of discharge by noting the goals that have been met, dropping subtle hints that discharge is not far away, letting them know that you are proud of their progress, discussing their discharge date days prior to actual discharge. All of this in order for them to accept what's going to happen ahead of time.

- Avoid the situation by setting clear goals during the initial evaluation, and making the patient aware that not only will they be discharged when they reach the established goals, but they will also be discharged if they DO NOT reach the goals in a reasonable amount of time because it would mean that physical therapy does not seem to be helping, and referral back to the doctor for a different type of interventions would probably be the best move. In this way, the patient is aware that exaggerating the symptoms will not contribute to their wish of remaining in physical therapy, so they won't do it.

- Tell them "I know you enjoy it here and I am glad we have made this a comfortable space for you, however we are not doing our jobs or providing adequate service for you if you are never able to fly on your own. Besides your insurance is going to kick you out soon if I can't justify services".

- Put the onus on the patient to help you help them. Go one on one with the patient and frankly tell them that you, as their physical therapist, want the best for them, and remaining in physical therapy for an indeterminant amount of time is NOT the best for them. The best thing for them is to return to their previous level of function.

- Use the "Mother bird" analogy, and make the patient aware that you, as a physical therapist, are like a mother bird preparing her baby birds (the patient) to fly. All you want is to see your patients "fly", so your reward is seeing them progress past the need for physical therapy, and your sense of accomplishment is directly related to the them getting better, and will be negatively altered if you are not successful in getting them back to their PLOF, and that is something that you do not want. If the patient has a heart, this may encourage them to get rid of the "physical therapy crutch, and take that step into independent functioning. As an added bonus, they may also feel too guilty to attempt to exaggerate their symptoms because they don't want to hurt you in the process.

- After taking final measurements, discuss the fact that they are almost ready for discharge, but let them know that you will be giving them an extra couple of treatment sessions before discharge so that you can be sure they are independent with their home exercise program, and to also allow them to prepare for it. This eases the discharge transition.

- If the patient is clearly ready for discharge, don't hesitate to discharge them. Be firm. Be very nice, but don't give them a choice, because this would enable toe patient who has become emotionally attached to therapy to "create" a reason to avoid discharge. Remember, every minute that the patient receiving physical therapy without the need is a minute they are losing their own independence.

- In a very cheery manner congratulate the patient by using the phrase "we have reached all of the goals we set at on the first day, so you are ready for discharge". Then go over home exercise program and anything else that he/she will need to function independently post-discharge.

- If you are in an outpatient facility which offers after-care exercise program for patients who have progressed past the need for physical therapy but who could still benefit from an exercise gym, offer it to the patient, and explain the program to them. Patients love this because it gives them a chance to continue coming to the PT facility. However, you will find that it works for you too because it helps patents accept the end of physical therapy, and eases your discharge.

How do I carefully tell a patient that physical therapy is not helping them, and they are not improving, and that other options may need to be explored.

When a patient comes to physical therapy, they are usually holding onto a hope that their problem will be taken care of, and that is usually what happens. However, there are times when after undergoing physical therapy, the patient does not improve. In this case the patient must be made aware of this. However, that is not always the easiest thing to do with a patient who is clinging onto the hope that we will "wield the magic wand" and make everything all better. This is especially true for the patient has exhausted a lot of other options, is in a lot of pain, or has multiple complex problems. The following are some helpful strategies.

- Be honest and say exactly that. Patients do respect honesty, even if its not what they want to hear.

- I do so by giving them a comparison of their objective findings on the initial evaluation as well as their progress report so that they can vividly see the lack of progress. Tell the patient that you have exhausted every option within physical therapy, and then discuss other options if you feel comfortable doing so, but let the patient know that you will be discharging them from physical therapy because it was not successful for them

- Tell the patient that, unfortunately, it is becoming evident that physical therapy cannot help them, and that it would be unethical if you told them anything else. Tell them what other avenues you recommend (MRI to gain more information on the cause, referral to another discipline, etc.).

- Let the patient see their progress in their own chart. Explain to them the meaning of things such as 4/5 strength versus +2/5 strength, Normal and abnormal ROM, and pain scale. Let them see with their own eyes that the improvement is not occurring. This makes it easier to explain the reason behind their lack of improvement.

- Simply tell the patient "We may need to refer you back to the orthopedic physician because conservative treatment is not helping".

- Make it easier on yourself by starting during the initial evaluation. At some time during the initial evaluation, state something similar to the following: "Physical therapy should help your problem, but if we don't see some significant improvement by the re-evaluation in 4 weeks, it probably means that physical therapy is not working for you, and we will then refer you back to your doctor to look at other means of
- addressing this problem". In this way, if the undesirable does happen, the patient is already prepared, and your job is easy. Simply remind them of what you discussed in the initial evaluation, and inform them that you will indeed be referring them back to the doctor for other means of addressing the problem as previously discussed.

- Make sure you try everything in your means to help the patient. Then go over, with the patient, every treatment strategy you used, the reason you chose it, and how it has failed to yield results. Then let the patient know that you have tried everything and are out of options. For example, let's say the patient came to you in outpatient setting with cervical radiculopathy and you tried everything you could think of including manual traction, mechanical traction, stability and ROM exercises, modalities for pain control, and postural training, but the problem never improved. Simply discuss with the patient how each of these interventions should but have not helped, and that you have exhausted all of your means of treating the problem, and rather than doing the same things over and over, its best to try something else besides physical therapy at this time.

- First, do a complete re-evaluation. Then inform the patient the things that has improved, the things that have not improved, and the things that are improving too slowly. Relate this to your decision to refer the patient back to their doctor, but most importantly, tell them what you will be recommending to their doctor (further medical testing such as MRI instead of x-ray, referral to pain clinic, referral to orthopedic surgeon, etc.). This will ease the patients mind knowing that even though physical therapy has not helped in this case, they still have options. The patient will also respect you for your diligence, and the doctor will be grateful for your input.

- Tell the patient the following: The reason your doctor referred you to physical therapy is to make you better. However, there are times when physical therapy does not help, and other methods of treatment may help instead. This appears to be one of those times. Since your progress is moving slower than acceptable, it doesn't make sense to continue with physical therapy because it is not helping. Instead of prolonging your pain and agony by delaying initiation of other options, it is best to let the doctor know so that he can act as soon as possible to get you started with another type of treatment option which may help.

- After first informing them that physical therapy is no longer an option, inform them that they may still have plenty of options, and then tell them that their doctor may have even more options. For example, if the patient has knee pain which is unresolved after physical therapy, tell them that there may still be options such as cortisone injections, surgeries which may or may not include knee replacement or less invasive surgery such as outpatient arthroscopic surgery, pain medications, or special custom knee braces. Tell them that the doctor may even want them to take supplements such as glucosamine or chondroitin which help repair knee cartilage. The most important part of this is to be clear when telling the patient that although these may be options, when they return back to the doctor, the doctor may have many more options that you have not even discussed. This gives the patient real hope for their future prospects, instead of allowing them to think that they have just wasted their time by having PT. It also makes for a well done job by the physical therapist even though physical therapy did not help the patient's particular problem.

- If the patient initially informed you that their doctor informed them that they are actually a candidate for surgery, but sent them to physical therapy in order to be sure that there was absolutely nothing else that could be done except for surgery, remind them of this during discharge so that they may be relieved in knowing that they have done everything that should have been done. If you know exactly which type surgery they will be undergoing, explain the general surgery and post-surgery rehab process to them. Be sure to include average length of hospital stay, what the incision scar will look like, how long rehab will take, etc.

How do I handle a situation with a patient who keeps disrupting my daily schedule because he/she is a chronic no-shower or is late very often?

This is one of the most frequent and frustrating situations that occur during the practice of physical therapy, especially in an outpatient setting. It is also one of the biggest indirect causes of problems for the new physical therapist. As a physical therapist, ample time is necessary in order to safely and competently practice physical therapy. Patients are usually scheduled systematically and in a way that allows the therapist enough time to treat and document in an orderly and efficient manner. However, when a patient shows up late, or not at all, this system is completely thrown off course. If you have two or more late shows in a row, it could get ugly. A type of cascading effect can take place. Patients treatments start to blend in with each other, some patients get angry, you don't have enough time to get documentation done and out of the way, you tend to rush treatment which decreases the quality of therapy, it looks to your boss/supervisor as if you are not efficient with your time if not incompetent, hazards and mistakes often occur during this time. And perhaps the most important thing of all...there is not enough time to think critically in treatment and planning, which substantially reduces the value of the said physical therapist. This is because a physical therapist is valued for his/her mind perhaps even more than physical attributes, and if the therapist has no time to effectively use the mind, he/she is of less use. All of this simply because a patient or two shows up late? The answer is yes. In short, it would not be wise at all to allow late patients to negatively affect your competence as a physical therapist. Here are some tips on how to deal with this problem.

- The patient will no longer get an appointment in advance. They can call the day of to see if we can fit them in at our convenience.

- Allow the slow patient to see that you have a patient waiting on you. Make sure they understand that the patient came on time, but you can't see them because your running now due to the slow patient. It may be enough to make the slow patient feel guilty enough about holding up another patient that they move a little faster.

- Let them know that their start and end times are firm and if they are late, their session still ends at the same time.

- Only allow the patient to schedule one visit at a time.

- Ask the patient "Are you having difficulty with transportation?" or "Do we need to change your appointment time? This allows the patient to get the message without you actually scolding them for constantly being late. If they continue to be late, show them the facility's cancellation policy they signed prior to beginning therapy.

- I charge them after the first no show, no exceptions.

- I always give one free pass/benefit of the doubt. If they are someone who is consistently late I will tell them that their time is just as valuable as the other patients who have appointments. It isn't fair to the other patients that the late patient is taking away from their time. They are usually understanding. If it continues to happen I will re-schedule them and charge a fee for the missed time. If they are truly horrible I will tell them they need to go somewhere else for therapy

- Make sure there is a full fee cancellation policy that automatically goes into effect if appt isn't cancelled 24 hours in advance except emergencies.

- Explain to the patient that you keep a schedule in order to have enough time to treat each patient effectively, and everybody wins if we all play our part and arrive at the scheduled time. But it is unfair to other patients when they are late because it takes time away from my other patients.

- Make sure they know and understand the no-show or late-show policy.

"Only allow this patient to schedule one visit at a time".
Venise Mule-Glass. PT,DPT,OCS,CSCS. Commack, NY.

- Tell the patient "I'm sorry, but I cannot see you anymore because you missed 2 appointments"

- Make sure they understand that you will be strictly following the no-show and late-show policy.

- Ask your supervisor if you could post the late-show/no-show policy in a prominent place so that all of the patients are forced to see it every time they come for therapy.

- If they show up very late 3 times in a row, tell them that you cannot treat them because it will take you away from other patient's time, and that will be unfair because they arrived on time.

- If there are other therapists who work with you, trade patients, and have the other therapist inform the patient that they arrived so late for therapy that you didn't have time to treat them.

- If you have an assistant, have the assistant treat the patient, and instruct the assistant to tell the patient that you are not very happy about them being late.

- If they arrive very late and it puts a strain on your time, cut the treatment intervention which they like the most. For instance, let's say that their POC calls for whirlpool for their foot, and exercise. If they really enjoy the whirlpool for their foot (as most patients do), skip the whirlpool for that day and just do exercise. They won't want this to happen next time, so it may help them to remember to be on time.

- Don't be a pushover. Let the patient see that you are visibly upset when they are late for their appointment. This will force them to take extra steps to avoid having to deal with you being upset with them at the next session.

How would I move a slower patient along faster so that they won't tie up all of my time, but without making them feel as if I am rushing them?

When dealing with a patient who does everything very slow treatment sessions can take longer than planned. This is not a good thing when your patient load is time-sensitive. It sometimes forces you as a therapist to juggle multiple patients at a time. And this, in turn, negatively affects you as a therapist in almost all areas directly or indirectly. It affects your decision making ability, patient safety, alertness, observational skills, and even your attitude and willingness to go the extra mile for your patient. Here are some very good suggestions on how to handle a situation somewhat similar to this.

- Use the power of touch by simply placing your hand on a part of their body such as a shoulder, their back, or hand and gently leading them into the desired direction while continuing to conversate with them.

- Tell the patient "I'm sorry, but I have a full schedule today and can only see you for ___ minutes", Let's see what we can fit in that time

- Do manual interventions first, then higher level therapeutic exercise second. After that, have them perform all lower level interventions with your PT Tech.

- Use a stop watch for their exercises. Instead of utilizing numbers of repetitions, utilize number of repetitions within a predetermined timeframe.

- Let the patient know that there is only so much you can do in a day, which means you can't complete a full treatment session, and part of their treatment will have to be delayed until the next session, which will slow down their progress. If they want their condition to improve in a reasonable time, they will move faster so that they can receive the whole treatment during each physical therapy session.

- While the patient is performing one exercise, prepare the next treatment ahead of time to decrease the waiting time. For instance, if the patient is riding the recumbent bike, and the next intervention is lying supine with moist heat on their back, while they are riding the bike get the moist heat prepared and have it sitting in place on the table so that as soon as the patient finishes the bike, all they have to do is lie on top of it.

- I would figure out what is taking them extra time and try to delegate the time to an aide to assist them or give them the responsibility to notify me when they are ready for the next step.

- Tell the patient "We have 45 minutes (or whatever amount of time you have available) to get all the treatment we can get in. Let's use those minutes as best we can".

- Adjust the bike seat and stand next to it visibly waiting for them to mount and start.

- If the patient has stopped moving or is moving slow because they are busy talking, dust off the treatment table and signal them with your hand to sit, while continuing to respond to their conversation.

- Hold the door open so that they understand that you are actually waiting for them to go through it.

- Gently move the body part into the desired direction, as if demonstrating. For example, if the activity to be performed is resisted shoulder flexion on cables, but the patient is moving slow because he/she is too busy reading and asking questions about an anatomical wall chart, place the handle in the patients hand and actually move the arm into flexion while carrying on the discussion about the wall chart. This is a good nonverbal cue that works well with patients who get preoccupied doing something else unrelated to the task at hand. It is also a good technique because it allows the therapist to progress the patient along without appearing as an impatient drill sergeant who keeps barking orders at the patient.

- If you are engaged in a conversation with the patient while they are moving too slowly, interrupt the conversation until they have done the activity you want them to do. For example, if the patient needs to transfer from the wheelchair to the bed but wants to finish making a point during a conversation between both of you, interrupt him in mid-sentence and say "lets first get you in the bed, then you can tell me the rest of it". Don't be afraid that the patient will think you are rude. Chances are that if they are "long winded", they already know it.

- Remember that in this kind of situation, you are the boss. You are ultimately in charge. You have a job that needs to get done for the benefit of the patient. And you are responsible for the care and improvement of the patient. So frankly tell the patient that they will have to pick up the pace. They are fully aware that you have a job to do, and will appreciate your honesty and the fact that you are only being diligent about your responsibility of helping them and you take your responsibility seriously.

How can I get the "talkative" patient to stop talking and start working without offending them?

This is a pretty common problem with patients who have been coming to physical therapy for a while. It usually starts off innocently enough. A patient may be performing his usual therapeutic exercises in the clinic such as riding a recumbent bike, for example, and then starts off a conversation with you. You, as the engaging therapist that you are, reciprocate. It becomes a very interesting and engulfing conversation. The patient stops pedaling for what would be a second or two in order to laugh or ask a question, but never resumes. The next thing you know, his 5 minute exercise has turned into a twenty minute conversation without exercise. Now, this was just for one exercise. Imagine how far behind you would be if the patient had ten exercises to do that day. This was just an example, and it shows that the patient has become comfortable with the therapy environment. However, most physical therapist have patients scheduled for appointed times, and do not have extra time on their hands for idle chit-chat with patients. It slows up their time, making the PT less efficient. It makes for a more hectic and stressful work environment because you don't want to offend the patient by saying "more work, less talk", so you tend to allow them to continue, and before you know it, you have three patients waiting for you at the same time. Here are some examples on how to avoid this problem.

- Refer to Question #10

- Tell the patient "I need you to focus on where you are feeling this exercise".

- Since it is impossible to talk a lot while breathing deeply and slowly, instruct the patient to "focus on taking slow deep breaths".

- Say," I don't want to be disrespectful, but we need to stay on track"

- Redirect to the task at hand. For example, say "I want you to focus on which muscles you are working right now". "Place your hand here on your leg just above your knee", "do you feel your leg muscles contracting when you kick your leg?". "Is this easy or hard?".

41

- "I'd love to chat right now, but I need to concentrate to help you right now".

- Keep talking, but use hand gestures to point to the next exercise immediately following the completion of one exercise. This way, you can sneak the next exercise in.

- "I have some questions that I need to ask you to be able to fill out your paperwork for the insurance company. Once we get them answered, I'll have time to answer your questions or hear you more on the topic".

- I will usually make a joke like "come on, you can move and talk at the same time.".

- Physically distance yourself from the patient while monitoring them for safety and proper performance of therapeutic exercise. This way, they can't get distracted with conversation because you are too far away from them to carry on a conversation

- Engage in the conversation for one or two minutes just to show that you are interested in what the patient has to say, but then say "hold on, I'll be right back" and leave. The patient should resume exercise as usual until you return. Return only when the patient should have finished the exercise.

- If you know this patient does this all the time, delegate the supervision to your aide or assistant while you address your other duties.

- Deeply engage in the conversation for an extended period of time, letting the patient hold you up. Allow the patient to see you get behind in you work duties. Then let them see how hard you have to work in order to catch up. They should feel bad enough to catch themselves next time as a courtesy to you.

- Carry on the conversation while constantly walking away to do something and coming back. Make sure that you walk far enough away so that the patient will eventually not be able to clearly hear what you are saying (make sure your assistant or tech keeps an eye on him/her while you do this). But don't stop talking. The patient will feel guilty about not performing his/her exercise while you are away, and start performing the exercises as he should be, but he won't feel as if you ignored him/her because you kept talking even though you were out of earshot of him. He/she will guess that you were simply unaware that he/she was not hearing you instead.

- I amuse the patient for a short while to let them know that I am listening, but then I say in a friendly way "hey, less talk, more work", and I point to whatever he/she is supposed to be doing. They usually get the point, shut up, and start performing their exercise.

- Continue engaging the patient in the conversation, but use hand motions to constantly steer him to perform the exercises. For instance, let's say the patient is supposed to dismount the back-extension machine, and mount the recumbent bike, but does not stop talking for longer than it takes to inhale enough air for the next five sentences. Since you can't get a word in edgewise, you can keep saying "yes" and "I see" while motioning for the patient to get onto the bike. You can also physical help the patient from one machine to the next if they won't allow you to verbalize the orders, it works well
- with elderly patients who frequently need physical help with transferring and transitioning from one exercise to the next.

- Jokingly say "More work and less talk". It will be funny, but they will get the message.

What can I do in order to get a non-talkative patient to open up and talk more?

Just as common as it is to have a patient who talks too much, there are patients who do not talk enough, especially about their particular condition. The reasons are too numerous to mention. Some patients are simply the "private type" and don't like discussing anything with a stranger about themselves. Some patients are the "strong silent type", are usually male, and don't like to discuss personal imperfections with others who may associate it with weakness. Some patients are just so nervous about being questioned about themselves by a stranger, that they don't know what to say. Regardless of the reasons, and for the patient's own benefit, we as therapists MUST get the information from them in any way possible. The following are some suggestions from other therapists.

- Ask the patient to describe to you what they are feeling at the moment during this procedure.

- Ask the patient to keep a journal on their smart phone regarding which daily activities elicit more pain, and which activities don't. Then discuss new journal entries at every physical therapy session.

- Find out their interests (family, hobbies, sports, etc.), then start a conversation about what interests them and correlate it with whatever information you need from them (subjective progress, HEP status, pain level, etc.).

"Ask open ended questions and give them adequate time to respond. Don't get uncomfortable with the silence".
Daniel Curtis, PT. DPT, MTC. Orlando, FL.

- First gather some personal patient data/history from the patient's chart. Then find something in which he is interested in, and try to start a conversation regarding that subject matter, and relate it to physical therapy.

- If you're a woman and your patient is a guy, ask him if he likes a particular sport (football, basketball, hockey, etc.). If he says yes, ask him to explain the rules of said sport. If you are a woman, he will be happy to open up and talk as he "teaches" you.

- Ask open ended questions… What are your thoughts about your pain? What 3 things can't you do that you want to be able to do? What do you do in your spare time? What do you like most about your work?

- Ask open ended questions and give them adequate time to respond. Don't get uncomfortable with the silence.

- Ask Avoid yes/no questions. Ask questions such as "How has this affected your life?", "Who will be helping you when you return home?", "What are your goals?", "Is there anything you feel we left out?".

- Place them in close proximity to other very talkative patients during exercise time in order to stimulate conversation. Patients generally love to tell other patients their story about how they ended up in physical therapy.

- Communicate the problem to them in a friendly, non-authoritative way to make them understand that it will make them get better faster.

- Let them see you talking very openly and friendly with another patient, and make the conversation seem very exciting and interesting. Then immediately go to them and try to strike up a conversation in the same manner.

- Be very blunt about it, and tell them that you need all the information you can get from them. Tell them the more info you get from them, the more you can help them.

- Tell the patient "the more information you can provide the better I will be equipped to help you".

- Don't scare them, but let them know in no uncertain terms that you will be doing a lot of things with them that may help them, depending on other specific factors being involved, and you need to know, otherwise without the info, things could go wrong, and you could possibly make things worse for them.

- Reward open discussion with positive reinforcement. Tell them that they are a good partner in their own recovery. Tell them that they are taking charge of their own future. Show

45

them that you are impressed with their openness, and wish other patients were as willing to share this type of vital information because it makes your job more effective and your life easier.

- Motivate the patient by telling them a story of how a former patient had great success when he/she was proactive in discussing their condition with you.

- Communicate the idea to them that you are only here to help, but you need feedback from them in order to determine if your help is working or not. Tell them that you can only do so much without information from them about their own body.

- Get the message across that nobody knows their body better than them…not even a physical therapist. So their active participation is necessary for improvement. Tell them that they need to tell you what feels better and what feels worse so that you can structure treatment that will benefit them the most.

- Use the phrase " you can't fix anything if you don't know how, when, where it is broken".

- Be honest with the patient and say to them " I know that you seem to not like discussing this, but if you can help me by giving me as much information as possible, I can help you by fixing the problem".

How do I handle an unproductive PT Aide/Tech?

Sometimes, as Physical Therapists and Physical Therapy Assistants, we find ourselves in a perfect situation where a therapy aide is exceptionally efficient, smart, eager to work hard and do a great job, and this makes us more productive. And other times, we walk into bad situations beyond our control such as starting a new job where our therapy aide is just simply lazy and works hard on avoiding hard work. This can make your job extremely difficult because not only are you doing the job of two people by doing the job they neglect to do properly, you are also being less productive, and your new boss may think your just not good at your job or with time management. It is unfair to you as a new therapist, but this scenario has been playing itself out in every PT facility every day in one way or another for many years. Here are some ways other therapist have successfully addressed this fairly common problem.

- Give them measurable tasks, and review them often.

- Educate and coach. Ask lots of questions and be clear about the productivity level. Check to see if your productivity level is reasonable and achievable. Be the aide for the day and see where the barriers might be.

- My belief is that through well-intentioned discussions, a lot can be solved. By showing to him/her what he /she could have done and what he/she actually did, we would discuss the ways that he/she could have achieved the goals. I would speak with honesty, professionalism but also with love and support. I would not forget to tell him/her that we are team and we want the best for our patients.

- Create a checkoff sheet that addresses their daily tasks and duties, then follow up through the day, making sure it is being utilized.

- Ask the PT tech how you can help them. For example, if they are not documenting as instructed, ask "are you having trouble with this documentation software? Can I show you some tricks to make it easier to use?".

- Discuss your expectations for them, and have frequent follow up meetings to discuss.

- Three things, communication, communication, and umm…oh yea, communication. Make sure you know what they expect, and they know what you expect.

- If you are sure that they understand your expectations, stick to it, no matter what. If you don't stick to what you say, the aide/assistant will assume that you are not serious, and then the problem will certainly worsen.

- In general, PTAs go to school for approximately two years, have a much higher knowledge base, and many have to take state board exams. So, they tend to take the job much more seriously than an Aide or tech who usually only have on-job training and can be teenagers or still in school for something else. So you must approach the two differently. A PTA may often seem lazy when they are just board with the humdrum aspects of their job, and want to be challenged. If this is the case, challenge

- their manual skills, intervention skills, or knowledge base. Then reward them when they prove their worth. You may find that this may light a fire under them. On the other hand, techs/aides may act lazy simply because they are. In this case, you may need to pull them aside and make them fully aware that you will not tolerate this type of behavior. Nine times out of ten, they already knew it was coming anyway.

- Sometimes, the PTA/tech may simply think you are abusing your position and insulting their intelligence with menial tasks. If this is the case, make sure that whatever it is you ask an aide or assistant to do, you can and will do yourself if necessary. Explain to them that you need them to do these things so that it will free up your time to do other things that they are not able to do.

- Give the aide/tech a few chances to choose to do their job instead of being lazy, and when they choose unwisely, stop what you're doing (if possible) and do it yourself. Make a mental note or write the incident down to remember it if need be. Then, after you have specific examples to refer to, explain to your aide/tech how inefficient and ridiculous it was for you to stop doing what you are doing to do their job. If patients had to wait because of the incident, bring it up, and tell your aide/tech that this will not be acceptable anymore.

- Don't ride your aide/techs back. Let them see that you respect their age and intellect, and expect them to do the right thing without constantly looking over their shoulder. Give them freedom to exercise good judgement when performing their job. Reward them when they show real responsibility by backing further and further off of their back and allowing them the freedom they desire. Then if this freedom is abused, let them know that they had a good thing going, and if they don't straighten up, you will be forced to treat them like they are younger than they are by constantly looking over their

shoulders making sure they do things right or micromanaging them. If they value
- the freedom to perform their job in a stress-free environment, and if you did indeed afford them the necessary freedom, they should straighten up fairly quickly.

- Get them alone and tell them you will give them one more chance to do things right. Otherwise, you will be dragging them (figuratively speaking...not literal. No, I mean it, not literal) into the office to report them. And if they defy you, then simply do it.

How do I delegate tasks to an assistant who is much older and has much more experience than me, without appearing offensive?

Situation: you (the new PT) ask your PT tech (who has been an employee for 4 years, and is usually an excellent PT tech) to put moist heat on a patient, and the tech not only questions your level of knowledge, but refuses to do it because "the other PT usually uses ice, so you must not know what you're doing". You ask yourself what just happened. Relax, this scenario plays itself out in just about every occupation in America, so why should physical therapy be any different. There are some who believe that in the job setting, the new guy is less qualified than the veteran guy to delegate tasks and instruct others to perform duties related to the job. Some may feel that you have to "pay your dues", "gain experience", or "earn the right" to give orders before they will take orders from you. This can be especially true if the person you are delegating a task to has worked there for much longer than you and/or is much older than you. Although this is a major concern with a lot of new PT graduates, it does not have to be a problem. Consider these things if you find yourself in this situation, and trust me, you probably will at some point in your career.

- Speak in a normal, non-derogatory tone.

- Approach this situation from a team perspective. When you ask your tech to perform a task, let them know that you will be performing another task at the same time. Your PT tech will realize you are simply performing your role on the team, not being a disrespectful idiot. They won't want to be the weakest part of the team, and will want to fulfill their role on the team by accomplishing the tasks that you delegate to them.

- Tell the PTA **WHAT** needs to be done, allow the PTA to determine **HOW** it is to be done, and let them know you are available for questions.

- First, remember that you have "earned the right" by completing years of higher education and by passing your board exam. Delegating work to others is an integral part of your job, so you should not be timid when performing that part of your job. If you delegate a job duty to a person, and it is refused, that person is in the wrong, and not you. Be fair when addressing the situation, but keep in mind that you are doing what you are paid to do.

- Just be professional. Don't get angry and start arguing with the person. That is the quickest way to lose credibility and respect. If it is urgent, and there is no time to have a side bar conversation with the person, do it yourself, and then (and this is a must) talk to the person in private.

- To avoid the problem at the start, be sure to delegate all tasks fairly regardless of age or job seniority. Chances are that the person just wants to be treated fairly, and is worried that your lack of experience will lead to lack of fairness. Making sure the person is aware of your ability to maintain fairness may completely eliminate the problem before it even starts.

"Make a list and give to the assistant and let them know you are available for questions". Kim Braun, PT. DPT. Beaverton, OR

- They have valuable experience that may be beneficial, so simply and honestly ask their opinion.

- It is generally not a good idea to tolerate insubordination because the problem will progressively worsen until it grows into a situation that is out of control. Address the problem immediately if possible, by asking the person to privately voice any concern they may have with your instructions to them. However, make it clear that you would otherwise expect them to follow your instructions.

- Remember that you are not god. We are all human, so we all make mistakes. If your instructions are ignored, don't ask the person silly questions such as if they went to school as long as you did, or try to be cute and say things like "let me see your PT license, oh that's right you're not a PT". It only makes you look like an idiot, and confirms their suspicions that you really are not qualified to delegate duties to others. Instead, first find out why your instructions were ignored. Maybe they simply forgot. Maybe they noticed something that you did not noticed, after all, they do have more actual experience than you. Even though they may have been wrong in their assumptions, maybe they truly thought they were doing the right thing in attempting to avoid harming the patient. The point is that you don't know until you ask, and you also cannot take action until you have all the facts.

- At the first sign of a problem, quietly and without making it a really big deal, pull the assistant to the side and tell them that you noticed some friction between the two of you. Tell them that you want them to be happy, and ask them if there was anything you can do to make your working relationship even better. If you use this approach, you avoid challenging them into what they may perceive as a confrontation. They may then view you as a class act.

- Get to know the people who help you do your job, and help them get to know you as soon as possible after you start the job. This will allow them to see you for the intelligent and professional clinician that you are. They will be more willing to accept your judgment calls without hesitation.

How do I convince patients to really listen and respect what I have to say, even though I am a new grad and appear young and inexperienced?

As a young and newly graduated physical therapist, you will encounter patients who are not comfortable with your skill and knowledge level because they simply believe a new physical therapist lacks the necessary level of competence. They may not consider your perspective or opinion as valuable as a more experienced and older physical therapist. This scenario is not due to any fault of yours, but if this problem is not overcome, it may decrease or limit the effectiveness of your interventions. So, it is your responsibility to you do all you can to help the patient realize that their assumptions of your lack of competence is unfounded, to say the least. Here are some suggestions.

- Speak in technical terms. Wear professional attire. Speak slowly and clearly.

- Whatever you do, DON'T SAY UHMMM!

- Always maintain professionalism. Remember that even though your clinic, office, or gym may be a fun place to work, your patients are not there for fun. They want to get better, and if they think in any way that you are not taking their recovery seriously, they will not take you seriously.

- Never argue about what is best for the patient. First simply listen to their concerns, explain the facts to them, then tell them what your OPINION is, and the best way to handle it.

- Respect is something that is earned. It will happen over time as you build a rapport with the patient and as they realize that their condition is improving.

- You have already graduated graduate school in Physical Therapy, so you KNOW what you're talking about. You know your stuff. However, make it a priority to take lots and lots of continuing education courses (suggestions are elsewhere in this book). In this way, you can be CONFIDENT that you know what you're talking about. Your own confidence in yourself goes a long way in translating into a patient's confidence in you.

- Listen to the patient's conversational tone, then speak in a tone relevant to that patient. For example, if your patient is an 80 year old arthritis patient who has an extremely light voice, speak in a tone similar to hers. Conversely, if your patient is a 19 year old shoulder dislocation patient who speaks in very loud tone, speak in a tone similar to his.

- Quote research studies that are relevant to the patient's problem, and then inform them you're your plan of treatment will be based on the successful treatment plans in the research studies that you quoted. Since this patient respects physical therapists with experience, they will respect the research study because they know that it was likely conducted by experienced physical therapists, and since your treatment interventions are based on the experienced researcher's findings, they will indirectly grant that same respect to you.

- Don't be afraid to touch your patient. The power of touch should never be underestimated in its potential to invoke empathy and respect. A light touch on the shoulder of a distraught weekend warrior who has just been told by you that his weekend basketball days may be over for the summer because of the knee injury, or a firm shake of a 70-year-old male hip replacement patient's hand can make a big difference in earning a boatload of respect.

Are there any time management strategies on how to effectively treat two or more patients at the same time without compromising quality of care?

This is one of the most often asked questions by new physical therapists. More often than not, new PTs find themselves working in a high volume physical therapy facility where they are constantly required to see multiple patients either simultaneously or in rapid succession. This scenario can make it very difficult for a physical therapist to perform his/her job duties in a sound and effective manner. It can force the new PT to rush, making it easier to make bad decisions and mistakes that they otherwise would not make. Needless to say, this kind of scenario can be a source of tremendous frustration, especially for the new physical therapist. Rest assured that this is nothing new in the world of physical therapy, so physical therapists have devised many remedies over time. Here are a few ideas that may help you.

- Try to treat both in the most open space available. This way, you can monitor one patient while treating another patient.

- Stagger their treatment times to start every 15 minutes, and immediately start with any one-on-one treatment. Then start them on modalities or exercise while you start one-on-one treatment with the next patient, and so one.

- Perform manual therapy on the first patient while observing other patient perform low level therapeutic exercises.

- The key is being able to multitask and have a good plan of care for both patients. You must take advantage of the patient that needs one on one time as the other patient may be on passive modalities. Making sure that they understand and can perform their exercise programs with minimal guidance in their progressions to insure best practice

- **The Rotating Phases technique.**
  If you have two patients at the same time, and they both need unattended e-stim and ultrasound, set up one one e-stim first, and then do the ultrasound with the other while the first patient is receiving ultrasound. By the time you finished with the ultrasound with the second patient, the first patient should be almost done with e-stim. Then reverse the order and place patient number two on e-stim while you do the ultrasound for patient number one. In this way, even though your treating two patients at a time, you will actually be providing one-on-one treatment for each of them during the same 30-minute interval. The same can be done with three patients at the same time (mainly in outpatient setting). The basic principle is to have all three patients receiving a completely different type of treatment at the same time, and then rotating the order one at a time. For instance, one patient can be receiving moist heat with electrical stimulation, while another is performing therapeutic exercise, and the third is receiving ultrasound treatment from you. Believe it or not, it can actually be done with four patients too (if you have an aide PT tech). The same would apply as above, plus you would have your aid/tech doing an ultrasound while you are performing manual therapy

or one-on-one interaction of some sort with the fourth patient. The key to doing this successfully is to make sure all phases of treatment are of fairly equal length of time (15 min for e-stim, 15 min of therapeutic exercise, 15 min of ultrasound including setup time, and 15 min of one-on-one interaction such as manual therapy of home exercise instruction). The other key is to be diligent in making sure the patients move to the next phase of treatment (rotate phases) within the same general time period.

- While one patient is doing a task that requires less of your time and effort than you can work with another patient on other interventions such as manual therapy.

- If you know that you're running behind and will have to make one patient wait to see you because your still busy with another patient, stop what you are doing, excuse yourself from your current patient by telling them you need to let another patient know that you have not forgotten about them. Then go to the second patient and personally tell them that you are almost finished with another patient and will be with them very shortly. Then resume your treatment with the first patient in an expeditious manner. Both patients will understand, and should appreciate your honesty, and it will also give a major time cushion in which to work with.

- In an outpatient setting, never do the same modality to two patients at the same time. For example, if your double booked with three patients and each of them have electrical stimulation, ultrasound, manual therapy, and exercise on their plan of care, put one patient on e-stim, have your aide do ultrasound with the other, do manual therapy with the third. By the time you're done, there other two will be nearly done, so just simply switch the order of things, while your aide supervises the patient doing exercises, in this way, no patient needs to wait, and everyone is done in an hour or so.

- Work in an open space where you have direct line of sight with all of your patients at the same time. Start your hands-on manual therapy procedures with one, then to the other, then to the third, and so on. In the meantime, have the other patients continue with their exercises.

How do I deal with a patient who cries uncontrollably secondary to pain every time I treat them, but does not want to stop treatment?

This scenario seems to play itself out fairly frequently, but the root cause of the problem may vary significantly in each individual situation. In this case, if you find the cause, then you find the solution. Don't be quick to assume that they are simply crying because it hurts. There are countless reasons the patient could be crying. Let's say that their initial cause of injury was due to a MVA in which their family member was hurt more than them or even killed. Let's make it more complicated and say that your patient was the driver of the vehicle. In this case, in this case, the patient may be crying to ease the guilt that they feel for being the cause of another person's pain or death. This patient will need extra time during their treatment session for your personal touch. They may be perfect discussion about how a psych therapist or social worker can help them. Inform them that you can easily refer them to them to a competent mental health professional who can help them while undergoing PT. problem solved. The point is to first find out why they are in distress before assuming what may seem to be the obvious.

- Some patients ascribe to the "no pain/no gain" model of rehabilitation. Inform pt that sometimes pain is not necessary for improvement, and that their gain may actually be delayed by their pain. Explain to them that you may need to ease up or stop and try a different route to the same goal if intense pain persists.

- There are some patients who think of the therapist as "God". They don't question the physical therapists decisions or actions in the least. And they would never ever dare say the words "that hurts". These may be some of your best patients. They are sometimes the patients who follow your instructions to the letter, and who always show up to physical therapy sessions on time or even early. They want to make you proud of them. While this may all seem like heaven to the therapist, you must be proactive when this character type cries with PT interventions. This situation should be "nipped in the bud" immediately.

- Explain to them you need the to work as a team with you in providing the feedback to treatment. I often use the phrase "you're the meter/gauge and I'm the operator".

- Teach relaxed breathing techniques to the patient.

- If they are crying uncontrollably, stop whatever you are doing anyway. Take a break and just talk it out.

How do I deal with a patient who does not fully or properly participate in therapy session because of being distracted due to recent life changes?

Most patients who are under the care of a physical therapist ended up in the situation due to a very undesirable occurrence (motor vehicle accident, sport injury, chronic injury, etc.). In addition to the physical damage that these injuries place on the patient, there is usually some emotional and mental stress that accompanies the injury. For instance, the patient involved in a MVA may have lost the life of a loved-one during the accident, the sport injury patient may have to deal with the fact that he/she will never be able to play as well as before and have a difficult time dealing with the inevitable, or the patient with the chronic injury may be dealing with the prospect of losing their job because of poor performance due to the effects of the chronic problem. It would be wise to look at the whole picture when attempting to handle a problem such as this. Nevertheless, it helps to have some cheat tricks to make it easy to navigate through this problem. Here are some tips.

- Address the problem head-on. First make note of the first few smaller incidences and bring it up in light conversation that you did notice the distraction. Then as soon as it starts to become a significant problem, refer back to the first time you noticed the problem, let them know that you are concerned from a therapist's perspective that the problem is slowing their progress. Then suggest an alternative. Here is an example. Mr. Johnson brings in a study guide for the MCAT test he has to take at school next week. You notice him still pedaling for several minutes on the recumbent bike after the timer has sounded. You say something to get his attention and alert him to what's going on like "is that book that interesting?" or "uh oh, looks like I'm going to have to pay close attention to you" or even a friendly "ummmm, Mr. Johnson, are you with us"(if your PT/pt relationship allows). The same kind of situation occurs a couple more times, and you respond in the same manner. Then the patient does something more significant such as doing 5 times as many resisted back extensions on the back machine as you have instructed him to do, all while reciting information from his study guide for memorization. At this time, stop the patient and in a very friendly yet stern manner remind him of the previous few times and let him know that you cannot allow this because it compromises his safety and slows his progress. Give him the opportunity to take responsibility for his own progress by reminding him that you need him to play his part on this two man team. I use the phrase "PT time is PT time, everything else is some other time". They usually get the message.

- If the recent life changes are in the form of the death of a loved one, and their progress is slowed by day-dreaming, lack of enthusiasm, acknowledge their loss, but don't throw a pity-party for them. Don't feed into the patient's grief. Remind the patient that they are there to get better. Make them aware of the fact that their loved one would probably want them to get better as fast as possible. If you can't seem to break through, then talk to them about referring them to a good social worker or psych professional.

- Tell the patient that you are committed to helping them recover, but it only works if they are as committed as you are. Otherwise, physical therapy will not help them.

- If the problem is due to a break-up or divorce (which I have seen quite a few times), try to empower them toward independence. Try not to get into the specifics, but interact with them from a coach's perspective. Inform them that exercise is a great way to get over a break up. If they are bitter and seem to want revenge, let them use therapeutic exercise as a tool toward that goal. I have used the phrase "the best revenge is to live well, so let's get better so you can live well".

- Inform the patient that you have noticed the distraction, inform them that its really going to negatively affect their progress. Then ask them if they would like to put physical therapy on hold for a while until they are able to focus on physical therapy.

How do I deal with a situation during an initial evaluation where my nervousness is showing, and causing the patient to feel nervous and uncomfortable?

You have been in this scenario many times during your clinical rotations in PT school, but the difference between then and now is that when it happened during clinical rotations, the patient expected you to be nervous and knew there was a licensed physical therapy making sure you didn't mess up. However, this time, as a licensed physical therapist, your patient's expectations are much different, and any nervousness may cause them to be uncomfortably concerned. Further, the patient's discomfort will likely cause you to be even more uncomfortable, which will in turn, further decrease the patient's comfort level with you in a vicious cycle that may spill into subsequent future sessions and interactions with the patient until discharge. This is simply not the kind of physical therapy relationship that you want to have with your patient, so let's see what can be done to avoid this scenario.

- Pause the evaluation, and explain the situation to them. Most people are empathetic enough to understand, and will want to take it upon themselves to help you get through it. This will make you less nervous, and thus make them less uncomfortable.

- Before you get started with the initial evaluation, converse with the patient on a more personal level. Get to know them, and let them get to know you a little bit. This may be the best trick in the book for this type of situation, not only because it eases the patient's nervousness, but yours also. It also provides an opportunity for you to inform the patient what school you graduated from, your degree, and how hard the program was to get through. This may make the patient more empathetic and patient toward you. They may actually want help you get through the evaluation successfully.

- Take a moment to excuse yourself and collect your thoughts. Then re-plan your approach, and return refreshed and ready.

- Try to "gain some time" through a light discussion with the patient about something that has absolutely nothing to do with physical therapy, all while you try to slow your breathing and concentrate on relaxing. As the conversation proceeds, you will become more comfortable, and your nervousness will decrease significantly.

- Remember that confidence is something that develops over time as you achieve successes. Understand that as a new grad, it is perfectly acceptable and expected for you to need to research a technique or ask for a second set of eyes on a case if the situation warrants it. Also, remember that PTs of all ages and abilities request help and struggle with difficult cases. If you accomplish these three things, you may realize that there is no need for nervousness, and the nervousness will vanish.

- Admit that you are nervous and why. Most people are empathetic to the innocent plight of others, and will understand. In fact, if they understand that you are nervous, they often try to make it easier for you, by being more patient and offering encouragement.

Are there any proven ways to explain/discuss the POC with patient while appearing knowledgeable but without sounding too technical?

During an initial evaluation, it is important to explain what you plan to do and the reason for it. However, due to the fact that the human body is as complex as it is, it is sometimes hard to explain the patient's condition in terms that are understandable yet factual. If it is done in a way that sounds too technical, you risk sounding like an idiot who simply wants to show how much more he knows about the human body than the patient. If it is simplified in a way that is appears to insult the patient's intelligence, the patient may lose a lot of respect and trust in you as their therapist. This translates to major problems further down the road such as non-compliance which then slows improvement. This means your effectiveness as a physical therapist suffers considerably in the process. Here are some suggestions from other veteran physical therapists to help you navigate around this problem:

- Don't be too specific when discussing your plan of care during the initial evaluation. If you are too specific, the patient may lose interest, and will probably just nod their head while they tune you out eagerly waiting for the end of the session.

- Use general concepts instead. For example, you can say "we will be doing a lot of exercise to strengthen your muscles, some manual therapy to get your (whatever body part) moving without so much pain and difficulty, I'll give you some exercises that I want you to do at home as an adjunct to what we will be doing in the clinic, and we might be doing some other things depending on how you progress. We will re-evaluate your progress sometime between now and a few weeks and send a report to your doctor to let him know if your making progress or not, and then we will go from there. Any questions?"

"Physically get down on your patient's level while explaining technical things to them". Evie, PT. New York, NY

- Speak in a patient first language and use pictures and anatomical models to supplement your explanation and patient education.

- I use the phrase "something we call" when explaining a physical therapy term to a patient. For instance, plantar fasciitis is a complicated condition that can be explained in layman's terms. However, if you simply refer to it as "tissue on the bottom of your foot that is inflamed" when the patient is in a lot of pain and has been treated by their doctor, had imaging and has been referred to physical therapy for treatment, the patient may think you have overgeneralized their particular condition, possibly because you appear young and may not know what you're talking about. Simply adding the proper term and then explaining what it means adds credibility to your words while making it easy to understand. So, using the aforementioned example to explain the condition, I would say "You appear to have a condition in which the tissue in the bottom of your feet responsible for helping to maintain your arch is injured and inflamed. This is something we call plantar fasciitis".

- Utilize various phone apps that show 3D motion graphics of musculoskeletal or neurological injuries and conditions, and how they are treated. They really are very useful, and there are tons of them available. Download several of these apps on your smart phone, and be prepared to use them.

How do I keep a patient enthusiastic about therapy?

When a patient is not enthusiastic about therapy, a myriad of negative things can occur, and each negative occurrence can lead to a cascade of negative events that can snowball out of control. For example, the patient may not want to participate in therapy, for whatever reason, and thus become non-compliant. Your patient's non-compliance may correctly or incorrectly be correlated by your supervisor with your competence as a physical therapist. As your boss's confidence in your competence level decreases, so does his/her patience with errors that you actually do make. You, as the therapist, then feel bad and stop looking forward to coming to work. And who wants to be in that kind of situation? Of course this is a hypothetical situation, but the point is that when a patient is unhappy, things go wrong. Here are some things you can do about it before the snowball forms:

- Keep exercises functional to their ADLs, recreational or athletic activities

- Provide alternate interventions that have the same effect. For instance, if your patient needs to strengthen their triceps, and they are bored with performing triceps pull-downs, have them perform overhead triceps presses instead. Both exercises achieve the same goal of strengthening the triceps, but the

62

patient gets to try something they perceive as new and exciting by simply performing the same exercise in a different way.

- Set hard goals. Constantly track progress. Constantly point out the progress they have made through their efforts.

- Concentrate and encourage the small gains in areas such as ROM, swelling, strength, pain, gait, etc. This allows more frequent opportunities for the patient to be enthusiastic about their progress because these gains occur so frequently throughout therapy.

- Make sure the patient notices that you are enthusiastic about them. Frequently state your goals and positive expectations for them. Make them aware that you see a great future for them.

- Use positive reinforcement. When something positive happens with the patient make small celebrations by telling them they are doing good, patting them on their shoulder, or letting them know that you will be documenting the progress.

- Use terms like "good job", "way to go", " not bad", "I didn't know you had it in you", or "I knew you had it in you".

- Let them know that they are exceeding even your expectations by showing surprise when they are able to do a lot more functionally.

- Tell them that you will have to increase the intensity of their exercise in order to keep challenging them. Tell them that it is getting harder to keep up with them.

- Allow them to see you brag about them to other patients or other therapists. Let them know that they are your "star pupil".

- Use other patients as example of how far they can eventually progress to. If there is another patient who has the same condition, and has made considerable improvement, let your patient interact with them or at least explain to them that you expect nothing less from them.

How do I exude confidence toward a patient, even though I am a new graduate?

As a newly graduated physical therapist, it is perfectly normal to feel nervous and somewhat uneasy in your new working environment. This can sometimes be perceived by patients as a lack of confidence in yourself as a physical therapist, which may negatively affect your patient's trust in your clinical judgement. This is not the best scenario to find yourself in, and understandably so, because your patients will need to have complete trust in your clinical judgement for them to be an active partner in effectively treating their condition. This, of course, means that it is your responsibility to exude the appropriate level of confidence to your patient that will help build their trust in you as a physical therapist. Here are some suggestions from veteran physical therapists that may help you do this.

- Spend a lot of time educating your patient about their condition. They will be impressed with your knowledge base, and this will give you more confidence that you will then exude.

- As a physical therapist who has studied for many years, and has successfully met all of the markers that confirm your abilities, including graduating from one of the most rigorous degree programs in college, obtaining graduate and undergraduate degrees in the process, and passing your board exam, you are highly skilled and trained physical therapist, so show it

- Know your stuff, Know your stuff, Know your stuff. You will automatically be confident if you know what you're talking about.

- Concentrate on keeping it simple and concise instead of concentrating on trying to impress your patient. This will actually impress your patient.

- Keep a ready supply of reference material in your office area in case you need to quickly read up on something. You can then take comfort in knowing that you can tackle anything that comes your way because you have a wealth of information at your disposal.

- Try to show as much confidence as you can. If your patient sees that you are confident, they become more confident in you, and the cycle returns to you because you will then feel more confident in yourself.

How do I convince a patient to "suck it up/bite the bullet" and do what needs to be done even though it is extremely difficult, but without appearing as an unsympathetic tyrant?

As a physical therapist, you will undoubtedly come across patients who are easily deterred by the level of difficulty involved in their recovery. These patients may attempt to avoid the challenging parts of their therapy by making excuses that therapeutic exercises are too difficult to perform or that pain is too great to fully participate in therapy. The patient may even provide various other excuses for the same reason. If you allow the patient to succumb to these excuses, treatment may not be as effective, and full recovery may be delayed. So, your job is to neutralize the excuses, and help your patient face their fears in order to overcome them. Here are some suggestions from veteran physical therapist on how to do this.

- Treat the patient in the same open space as another patient who has had the same condition and same treatment, but has already progressed well with physical therapy. Allow the two patients to talk about their condition and let them compare notes.

- There are no cookie-cutter type of patients when it comes to tolerance to therapeutic interventions that are not very comfortable. Some patients have the no-pain-no-gain mentality, while others are completely terrified of pain and will do anything to avoid it. Here are some suggestions in navigating through the maze that is a patient's emotional tolerance to therapy.

- First talk to them and determine what makes them tick. Then use it to encourage and motivate them

- Use the term No pain-No gain if appropriate

- Let them see another patient who is working exceptionally hard and who is making visible improvement

- When they show courage, make it obvious that you are very pleased and even proud of them

How do I convince other veteran therapists to share their wealth of knowledge on a particular subject without appearing stupid?

You finished undergrad with honors. You completed graduate school with a 4.0 GPA. You were the student all of your former classmates went to for answers to questions during PT school. So why do veteran physical therapists know more than you? The answer is quite simple. They have knowledge gained by experience. There are two ways to attain their level of knowledge. The first method would involve you spending several years experiencing the same things they have experienced while making mistakes and errors along the way. The second method is to find a way to transfer their knowledge to you (I would suggest the second choice because it is the easiest and fastest). Convincing veteran therapists to transfer their knowledge can be a tricky thing to do. First, it puts you at risk for not appearing knowledgeable. Second, it may seem like an unfair trade to them because you get everything from them while they appear to get nothing from you except the knowledge that they gave you knowledge. Thirdly, who has time to spoon-feed some newly graduated PT. And lastly, some veteran PT's feel that since they have learned their valuable pearls of wisdom the hard way, you should too. With all of these obstacles, how is it possible to feast on some of the knowledge possessed by veteran physical therapists? Well here are some suggestions.

- First demonstrate that you do have some knowledge on the subject, then ask them to share their advanced knowledge

- If you don't know ANYTHING about the subject, then you must do at least a small degree of research before you go to the veteran Pt to ask for advanced knowledge.

- If you have the chance, watch how the veteran PT addresses the particular subject on their own during any normal day of work, and take notes.

- Let them see that you are thirsty for knowledge in all that applies to the practice of physical therapy, and then ask them to allow you to "bounce some ideas off of them".

- Making sure they understand that you are a new graduate, compliment their skill and technique, and ask if they would mind if you learned some things from them.

- Ask how long they have been in practice, and get to know how they got into PT, inform them that you are honored to work with such an esteemed veteran PT. After this, you should be able to ask them questions about anything because they will probably be more than willing to be part of your learning experience.

How do I stay awake while performing an ultrasound treatment?

Yes, this actually was a legitimate concern among new physical therapists that I polled. Apparently, the circular motion of the ultrasound transducer head elicits some type of relaxing/hypnotic response in the clinician that causes them to feel sleepy, especially if it's done during early morning hours. So, I asked experienced physical therapists who have been in the business for many years for their advice, and this is what they told me.

- Don't stay up all night before work

- Ask questions about things like the weather, and strike up a conversation

- Don't sit down while performing an ultrasound if your already sleepy

- Switch hands frequently

- Explain how ultrasound works and its benefits to the patient

- If your already sleepy, don't find a comfortable position for yourself while performing the ultrasound treatment

- If it doesn't bother the patient, whistle a lively tune during the ultrasound treatment.

- For me, coffee early in the morning is always an option

- Delegate the task to a PTA or PT Tech

I'd like to see some effective tips/advice techniques frequently used by other veteran physical therapists for patients at risk for injuries?

As a physical therapist, it is no secret that you are an expert in the field of musculoskeletal injury prevention. You are the "go to" person on the subject, so when people have the opportunity to get expert advice they take full advantage of it. The interesting thing is that over the years of practicing as a physical therapist, you will find that most patients repeat the same questions. As time goes on, you will learn to avoid providing lengthy explanations to the same questions over and over again to patient after patient. You will learn to answer these question in a very efficient, yet effective manner. But why wait when others have already spent the time to perfect these answers?

- "No pain-no gain does not apply to your particular situation".

- "Always stretch and warm-up before you do your sport/exercise activity".

- I remind older patient at risk for falls to clear all walk areas in their home and have grab bars installed in the bathroom.

- If they are a weekend warrior who constantly injures themselves, remind them that "they were lucky this time".

- If they are an older weekend warrior, remind them that they are not as young as they used to be, and healing time takes longer, plus repetitive injuries to the same body part may cause irreversible damage in the long run".

How do I deal with a patient who makes unwanted and inappropriate sexual or romantic advances toward me, whether overt or covert?

Believe it or not, this does happen more often than not. To understand why this happens, put yourself in the patient's shoes. Imagine if you had a kind and caring person who happens to be very knowledgeable physical therapist, and who spends a lot of time and effort tending to you in order to make you feel better. This person constantly fusses over your every discomfort and genuinely wants to make you happy. It's something we probably all want in a relationship. Now snap out of it because it's an unrealistic fantasy. First of all, make no mistake, it **IS** a job that you are doing. Secondly, although your treatment approach is individually tailored for that particular patient, it is not personal. And although the patient may be completely unaware of it, you may be doing exactly the same thing with the very next patient. Thirdly, the patient-therapist relationship is a fragile one based on mutual respect for the other's role. If you allow
yourself to be drawn outside of its fragile walls, you risk losing that respect and compromising your dignity. Saying this, I must also state the obvious fact that one does not want to be rude and insulting when politely refusing any inappropriate advances. This, of course, places the physical therapist in an awkward and precarious position. The following are suggestions on how to walk the thin line between responding with professionalism or responding with rude/insulting behavior.

- Have an assistant or tech with you and the patient at all times if you must treat them in a private or secluded area. Otherwise, never treat this patient in a private area.

- Act immediately. Understand that every minute you wait in dealing with the matter is a minute that the patient's hope increases. Thus, refusing the advances in the end it is that much more difficult for both of you.

- Acknowledge and confirm that it is indeed inappropriate advances before you begin to turn them down. Otherwise, it could get a little embarrassing when you are trying to reject advances that the other person is not making.

- If the advances are very overt, simply say "listen, I am your physical therapist, so what you are saying (or doing) is completely inappropriate, and even indulging in that kind of conversation (or behavior) would be unprofessional of me. I am going to have to ask you to stop".

- In order to avoid hurting the patient's feelings, a little white lie may be necessary. You can tell them that you have a boyfriend/girlfriend. However, there are some who disregard this with the idea that they possess the ability to make you want to break up with your boyfriend or girlfriend. If the patient seems obnoxious enough to persist even after being told that you already have a boy/girlfriend, resort to the old "I'm married. I just take off my ring at work because I use my hands to perform massage and other manual techniques".

- In some states it is illegal, so make a call to your state's Physical Therapy Association to confirm for your state.

- Switch patients with another therapist if you work in a setting with multiple physical therapists.

- Be very serious and completely honest with the patient. Tell them that you take your job and career very seriously, so their proposal would be out of the question.

- Refrain from saying things like "I'm sorry but you're not my type" or mentioning the phrase "I'm flattered" at all in this situation. It sends mixed messages, and gives the listener the idea that there is still a chance that they can change your mind.

- Tell the patient that you simply don't date patients or former patients (in case they return after discharge). This seems to work well, while highlighting your professionalism.

How do I deal with a situation where I am romantically interested in a patient?

First of all, after reading #27, one should understand that this type of situation is a very difficult one to answer. It should be understood that all recommendations here are simply suggestions from other therapists. I have found that many therapists think of this scenario differently. There are some therapists who initially met their spouses when their spouse was there patient. There are also Physical Therapists who believe that once a person is a patient of yours, that patient-therapist relationship never ends (even after discharge). However, NONE of the therapists polled believe that the active patient-therapists relationship should be compromised. Ultimately, it is up to you to maintain the strict code of conduct which is becoming and expected of the professional that you are and the profession that you represent. Consider the following suggestions from your esteemed colleagues:

- If the patient has not been discharged from your care, consider the suggestions in #27 and reverse the roles, but keep the rules.

- If you find the urge to cross the line of professionalism is too great, transfer the patient to another physical therapists care before you act on those urges.

"PT/Patient romance is on the other side of a line that is not to be crossed" Giselle Defreitas, MPT. Washington, DC.

- Whatever you do, do not even discuss the remote possibility of a romantic connection while the patient is still under your care.

- Don't even think of attempting to carry on a secret affair with your patient. You WILL get caught, and it will get out to other staff members. Rumors will spread, and after the rest of the staff discovers what's going on, you will lose every drop of professional credibility that you had earned up to that day. You might as well start looking for another job because it will probably get worse from there, not to mention the fact that you could get fired.

- We are all humans, after all, and there are times when our emotions seem too powerful to control. If this is the case with you and your patient, continue to avoid discussion about a romantic connection, but make a single subtle hint that after they are discharged from your care as a patient, it would not be considered very unprofessional if the two of you "went on a date or something".

- If the idea of getting to know the patient outside of work is so appealing to you that you cannot contain yourself from approaching them outside of work, at least transfer them to the care of another therapist first. It's not pretty, but at least the patient/therapist relationship is left intact.

- Whatever you do, do not pursue. Period. End of story. Don't do it.

- Do not pursue until the patient has been discharged from physical therapy, and speak to them on their way out of the door, but do not get their number from their chart and call them, because that's creepy.

- If you feel that you may have already compromised any professional codes, don't find a reason to make sure that patient is treated by another therapist from that point on, and avoid the patient like the plague. Gather your courage, summon your inner strength, and apologize to the patient in private, telling them you may have been inappropriate. Then simply remind them that for as long as they are your patient, you will not behave in any way except as appropriate for a physical therapist in relation to their patient.

How do I deal with a patient who does not take Physical Therapy seriously?

So, you explain home exercises to your patient, and during several of the patient's subsequent PT session, you ask how the exercises went, only to hear that they didn't have time to do them or simply forgot. Or let's say your patient repeatedly request that you modify your treatment interventions in order to speed up their therapy session because they have other things to do and places to go. Or how about when you catch your patient lying and cheating himself/herself out of exercise by telling you that they "already did the third set"? Although not always the case, these things are a red flag that the patient does not take physical therapy seriously. A patient who thinks and behaves this way can be very difficult and unpleasant to deal with, and because they are not keeping up their end of the deal, they can actually decrease the effectiveness of your efforts to resolve their condition.

- Always make sure he/she understands that you take it seriously.

- Immediately address any instance where the patient demonstrates lack of interest. For example, at the first sign of patient non-compliance with HEP, first explain the benefits of the home exercise program, then be very professional but straightforward when explaining to them that you have taken the time to structure a HEP for his/her benefit. Ask them to let you know if they do not intend to take PT seriously because your valuable time can be spent with many other patients who need your help.

- First make sure you have tangible rationale that reasonably validates your conclusion that the patient doesn't take PT seriously. For example, they admit to repeatedly being non-compliant with home exercises. Then call the referring physician and inform them that you will be discharging the patient and why. Then discharge the patient while not forgetting to highlight the rationale, and refer them back to that doctor for further explanation on the reason for their discharge.

- Politely ask them why they seem to be taking their own health and recovery so lightly. You can say in a friendly tone, for example, "I noticed you seem to be taking this very lightly. Do you want to get better? Because if you don't really care, we should stop at this point".

- Tell them that you regularly inform the referring physicians how enthusiastic and compliant the patient is. This sometimes makes the patient realize that their actions are being monitored, so they may tend to get more serious.

I need veteran therapist-approved tips for taking a really good history?

I am certain that all of your professors and clinical instructors have repeatedly hammered into your head the idea that taking a really good patient history is one of the most important parts of Physical Therapy Evaluation, so there is no need for me to beat a dead horse here. However, I do know that taking a good history is sometimes easier said than done. Getting the patient to volunteer the right information is sometimes like pulling teeth. Some patients may give tons of information, but very little of it is useful, while others may give useful information, but they give very little of it. Sometimes, using well-chosen phrases can make the lightbulb come on in their mind and make all the difference in causing the patient to give you the most useful and relevant history in the most efficient manner. Here are some of the phrases various physical therapists use regularly in order to obtain the most appropriate past medical history from patients:

- "any other medical problems?"

- "has anything like this ever happen to you before"

- "any broken bones, surgeries, or physical therapy in your past?"

- "have you ever had physical therapy before?"

- "When did this happen?"

- "Have you ever had physical therapy in the past?"

- "How long has this been bothering you?"

- When and how did you get injured?

- Did you have immediate pain after this?

- What did you do next?

- Did you have an x-ray and MRI taken? If so, why did it say?

- Did you try anything prior to seeking physical therapy?

- Have you had physical therapy in the past?

- Is this the first time you had this type of injury?

- Is it worse a certain time of the day.

- What are you doing when it feels better versus when it hurts the most?

- Any numbness or tingling noted?

- Remember "5 Ws and an H" (who, what, when, where, why, and how).

How do I tell a person that part of their problem is the fact that they are overweight, and that they need to lose weight, but without offending them?

There is no need to state how difficult it is to navigate through this situation, especially when the patient is a woman. For various reasons in our society, a person's weight is deeply connected to their sense of self-esteem. It is a topic that can evoke strong negative emotions from the patient, and these emotions can range from feeling insulted, ashamed, or even embarrassed. This, in turn, can make you very uncomfortable and reluctant to provide important information to the patient for fear of making them feel even worse, which may then decrease your effectiveness as a physical therapist. The whole thing has all of the makings of a very complicated lose-lose situation, but it doesn't have to be this way if you equip yourself with the right tools when you approach the scenario. Here are a few tools for you.

- Cite studies that clearly and objectively demonstrate the negative repercussions of the weight, and the need to lose weight.

- Just come right out and say it. Believe me, they already know. They won't feel insulted, and will and respect you for being honest even though it may make them feel embarrassed.

75

- Ask the patient to imagine how much hip/knee/ankle pain (whichever joint is involved) they would experience if they walked around with a heavy backpack on. Then ask them to imagine how that joint would feel if the took the backpack off and walked around without it. Make the connection to their excess weight, and they should get the picture.

- Ask them to walk while carrying a 20-lb. dumbbell and tell me how it affects their chief complaint. Then have them walk without it and ask them how that feels. They will get the point.

- Actually, take the time to calculate their BMI for them, and them explain to them what it means regarding their condition.

- Using objective measures of health such as BMI, explain to them how excessive loads negatively affect the joints, movement, etc.

"Discuss the positive vs negative effects of excess weight in an objective way, as it relates to conditions similar to that of the patient's". Natalie Maharaj, MPT. Annandale, VA

- The patient is already fully aware of the fact that their weight is part of the problem, so you don't have to tell them. Instead, give them hope by relating positive stories of patients who have improved after losing weight.

- The most important thing is to be frank with the patient from the time you first meet. After that, informing her/him that weight is exacerbating her/his problem is much easier and less awkward.

- Make sure you are in a private area in the clinic, and say something similar to " I need to be brutally honest with you, and that I don't wish to offend you, but part of the problem is excess weight.

- First explain the diagnosis, and then enumerate a list of things which make it worse. If excess weight is one of those things, then include it in the list with the other items.

How do I prevent documentation/work duties from forcing me to stay late after work in order to catch up?

Catching up on documentation is the number one reason physical therapists stay late after work. As the social butterfly that you are, you have things to do and people to see, so you don't have time to hang around at work when you are not getting paid to do so. There are only so many hours in a day, so take note of some of the things you can do to avoid spending them at work unnecessarily.

- Three things: Document as you go along. Document as you go along. Document as you go along

- Don't leave things undone from the previous day because that just means there is more for you to squeeze in on the following day

- Don't treat more than three patients consecutively without completing all of the documentation from those patients

- Document during down time

- Although not advised because it may become habit forming and cause regret later, if all else fails, document during lunch.

- If it's because of a slow patient, refer to the elsewhere in this text book

How do I deal with a person who constantly tends to overdo the exercises I have prescribed?

As a physical therapist, you will run into this patient sooner or later, and then will see this type of patient again and again throughout your career. They are almost always very nice people, but often cause exacerbation or further injury to themselves by repeatedly attempting to increase the intensity level of the exercises that you prescribe to them, slowing down their own progress, and becoming a source of unnecessary frustration to you as their physical therapist. Simply telling them to avoid overdoing their exercises has little to no effect on their actions, and they often unfairly blame you for the delay in their progress, eventually. It would be very wise to have a strategy for this patient. Lucky for you, other physical therapists have already created strategies that you can adopt, and here they are.

- Explain overuse injuries with the patient. Sometimes, being informed makes all the difference.

- Discuss with them that more is not always better, and how overdoing things can hinder progress.

- Ask your patient to think of their exercises like pouring a can of Pepsi. If you pour too quickly into a glass, more foam develops (pain and re-injury) and you actually don't get all of it in the glass until the foam subsides. However, if you pour it slowly into the glass minimal foam (pain and re-injury) develops and you actually are able to pour all of the Pepsi into the glass at once. Exercise is just like that analogy. If doing it appropriately you can get much better and quicker results versus doing too much as your body will not have enough time to heal and increased inflammation can occur.

- Use the expression, "a cup of ice cream is good to your stomach, a gallon of ice cream gives you a stomach ache".

- Explain that you are a very competent physical therapist who will deliver the very best treatment possible in order to attain their goals. However, strict adherence to exercise instructions is necessary to accomplish the goal, and so you will not continue treating him/her if they are not compliant with your precise exercise instructions.

- If you are convinced that the patient will hurt a lot after relatively light exercises, and the patient doesn't think so, allow them to do just enough exercise while under your direct supervision so that the pain will get his/her attention and make them understand that progression needs to be gradual.

- Make sure the patient understands the purpose of the exercises you have prescribed.

- Go over the proper performance of the exercises with the patient in order to make sure they actually understand how to perform them.

How do I deal with an aide/tech who does not respect my authority?

This is apparently a common problem, especially with new physical therapists, and especially if the e34therapists is younger than the tech or the tech is a long-time employee of the facility in which the two now both work. The new therapist is sometimes viewed by the tech as "unproven" or not yet worthy of receiving a high level of respect. There are times when the tech has worked for a long time with the therapist whom you are replacing and may have developed an emotional bond, and now resents you as the cause of their loss. There are instances when the tech was allowed to disrespect the PT before you were hired, and simply expects things to remain as they were. Sometimes, it's just a matter of the tech being very unprofessional. And still, there are instances where the problem is that the tech simply has a personality which clashes with the therapist's personality. The causes of the problem are too many to list here, but the important thing to remember is that there IS a reason for the problem. All you have to do is investigate and find out what that reason is, then be creative and act accordingly. Here are some ideas from other therapists that may help you in this type of situation.

- Even though the tech may be wrong, mutual respect must be shown on both sides. And since you are the party with the most authority, when there is a stalemate, it sometimes means you will have to be the first to offer a display of respect.

79

- Make sure that your own actions are respectable. Make sure they see that you always follow the rules yourself.

- Don't fraternize a lot with your techs, especially if they are not very respectful.

- Find a clear incident where the tech is being disrespectful to your authority, and immediately pull them aside and find out why this is happening. You can start by saying something like: Jane, between me and you, I noticed you giving me a hard time with this or that, and its making it difficult for me to do my job. What's going on, Jane?

- Make sure that your techs/aides have a clear understanding of what you expect of them.

- Always address any problems immediately. Never let the problems multiply or snowball. If this is allowed to happen, it may be too late to correct the problem.

- Although the power of authority can be intoxicating and easily abused at first, just remember that although you are a therapist, you are not God. So be respectful of your
- techs/aides as you would like them to be respectful of you.

How can I make physical therapy a fun place to be for me and my patient?

Although we as physical therapists absolutely love our jobs, and wouldn't even think about having any other occupation, the work can sometimes seem repetitive, and this makes the day feel longer. Even the patient can feel this way, especially when you consider that they physically work harder than you do during their PT session, and are usually in some sort of pain. When your spirits are down and you don't feel so great,
your patients tend to pick up on it and feel the same way. You then pick up on their feelings, and complete the vicious cycle by feeling worse, yourself. This makes for a very bad day for you and your patient, and both of you end up wishing you were somewhere else. Here are some suggestions on how to avoid this

situation:

- Start with yourself. Make sure you are being cheerful and fun.

- Always have good music playing in the background

- Get to know your patient on a more personal level

- Strike up conversation with patient about anything while you're doing your job

- Think of good jokes to say and try them out on your patients

- Play practical jokes on your co-workers during down time (sew a string of thread to a dollar bill and stealthily place the bill in a conspicuous place on the floor where everyone can see it. Yank it away every time someone stoops down to pick it up. Just make sure they can take a joke first. This one always kills 'em).

How do I convince other therapists to help me with my patient load when I am overloaded, but without appearing as if I cannot pull my own weight?

There are times in any PT facility when a physical therapist could simply use a hand from another physical therapist in order to manage a caseload of patients. It's simply a very common situation that every therapist finds him/herself in sooner or later. It also has no bearing on the person's capabilities as a physical therapist. However, when a newly graduated physical therapist joins a PT staff, there is sometimes bias against the perceived level of competence and capabilities of that new physical therapist. And when the new physical therapist finds himself/herself in a frustrating situation which requires help from other therapists on the staff, others may view it as resulting from the new therapist's incompetence. It is unfair, but you as a new therapist do not want to add to this unfair yet very real bias. These suggestions should help ease your transition into your new position.

- First make sure you help other therapist staff members out as often as possible when they need you. In this way, when you need help from them (and you eventually need will), they will remember when you helped them, and not be so quick to label you as incompetent.

- Be straightforward and ask, but only when it's absolutely necessary. Don't abuse the privilege

- Show them that it is in the best interest of the patient.

- If you are overloaded with patients or behind with notes, then ask someone if they can cover a patient so you can catch up. Just remember to offer to help them when your schedule slows down too. It's all about teamwork.

"Insist that you be allowed to manage your own patient appointments". S. Marley, MHS, PT. Washington, DC.

- When alone with the other therapist, let them know that you want to pull your own weight, but are still gaining experience and learning, but you don't want you make your patients suffer while you learn. Ask them to feel free to let you know if you seem to be asking for help too much.

- Ask the other therapist to feel free to ask for help from you when you need it.

- Try to avoid the need for help from others by maximizing your time management skills (see elsewhere in this text for help).

- If you find yourself in a situation where you need help, don't leave it up to the helper to determine exactly how to help. Decide exactly what the other therapist needs to do in order to help, and instruct them to do only that thing.

82

- Make a "friendly favor agreement" by telling the helping therapist that you will return the favor the next time they need help. Tell them "you owe them one", and then make sure you fulfill your promise as soon as possible.

- Frequently offer your help to your fellow physical therapy staff-members. Become known as the therapist who is always very eager to help others. This way, other therapists will be more willing to help you.

How do I negotiate a decent salary as a new grad even though I have almost no experience?

It's no secret that a new physical therapist will not be able to demand the same amount of salary from a prospective employer as a veteran PT. However, you should NEVER settle for less than what you are worth when it comes to negotiating a salary. This presents a difficult problem for new physical therapists because the prospective employer has the advantage against your claims of being worth a higher salary based on your inexperience.

- If you have decent grades, make sure you inform your potential employers. Tell them that your grades during physical therapy training are an excellent expression of your overall potential as a physical therapist, and that you would like to be compensated accordingly.

- If your grades were average, don't concentrate on the grades. Instead, concentrate on your work ethic, personality, people skills, punctuality, professionalism.

- To be honest, you really can't negotiate salary. If you are offered something a lot less, then you can always shop around, but if that's the place you really want to work, then take it because it may offer a lot more to make up for the lower salary (more time with patients, better mentoring program, better work/life balance, etc.). You could also ask that your salary be reconsidered after a 3-month probationary period.

- Agree to become certified in a particular specialty area by a specific time at no cost to the facility. Then hiring you brings value to the facility.

- Go online, and lookup average salary for physical therapists in your area. There are various sites. Find the site with the highest salary matching your area, print the info before you attend your interview, and show it to your potential future employer, only when the subject comes up (when they say "what kind of salary are you looking for").

- Ask the salary of friends who are working therapists. Ask them if you can use them to vouch for the going salary rate if necessary.

- If the salary offered is too low, ask "what can I do to raise this starting salary".

- Get reported salary ranges from five different internet sources, print them and refer to them. Just make sure they are within the range that you want.

- As early into the interview as possibly, let the interviewer know, in a calm and professional manner, that you are already considering several job offers.

- Tell the potential employer that of all the job offers that you are considering, you like their facility most. Tell them that you are close to accepting the offer, and probably would, but salary is just too low for you to consider it, but leave the door open for negotiation by saying "unless there is some other way to work this out".

I want to be viewed as the "therapist" and not the "new grad". How can I make this happen?

This appears to be a concern of many new physical therapists. Most veteran therapists seem to equate the idea of the "new grad" with the idea of the "immature therapist". This actually gives you a simple way to help resolve the problem, and that is to simply demonstrate maturity.

Here are some suggestions by other therapists on how to accomplish that task:

- Talk about all the new ideas which may not yet be well known, and that you learned at school.

- Don't place too much stock in how patients view you, as long as you are trying your best to be the best therapist you can be.

- Learn as much as you can and as fast as you can from other veteran physical therapists, and then emulate the best of what you learn.

- Limit any unprofessional conduct from your behavior, and don't associate with those who behave unprofessionally.

- Work hard to earn it and then demonstrate it.

- Use a firm clear voice when talking with patients and colleagues

- Be clear and straight to the point in your dealings with others

- Don't just get to work on time every day, be there earlier or even before anyone else. This is a hallmark sign of a professional.

- Dress the part. For example, if your uniform consists of a shirt and tie, realize that you are no longer a "starving student" and wear the best shirt and tie you can find. If it consists of scrubs, be sure they are ALWAYS ironed, they are clean, and tucked in perfectly.

- A clean-cut look never hurt anyone. NEVER come to work appearing as if you forgot to shave, or you woke up too late to do your hair.

- Always act in a way that your supervisor would use you as an example of how to conduct yourself at work.

Give me some veteran physical therapist-approved layman terms/phrases or techniques for explaining anatomical structures such as tendons, ligaments, joint capsules, etc.?

As a physical therapist, you are the unquestionable authority and expert in human physical anatomy, and part of your duty to your patient is to impart some of your knowledge on the subject to the patient relevant to their condition. However, if you do it in an awkward manner, it becomes difficult to understand, and you run the risk of giving the patient the impression that you are not fully informed. This can cause the patient to lose confidence in your ability to treat their condition, and things to can go downhill quickly. It's a good idea to have some "go to" phrases and explanations that are guaranteed to get the job done in the most effective manner possible. Here are some phrases that experienced physical therapists suggest using.

- Use the phrase "something we call" and then tell them what it means. It allows you to be specific and deliver the information, but yet use simple explanation for easy understanding. Here is an example: "The pain is caused by "something we call a bone spur", which is a build-up of bony deposits at the end of the bone which pokes into your soft tissue every time you take a step".

- Tendons are like duct tape attaching muscle to bone. Ligaments are like stiff rubber bands. Joint capsules are like plastic baggies around the joint.

- Tendons: Either a short of long extension of the muscle which is attached to a bone at the other end. The muscle pulls the bone by pulling on the tendon like a string. When injured, its usually called a strain or tear. A rope-like tissue that elastic enough to be able to be stretched when necessary, and strong enough to help move bones when needed.

- Ligaments: Very strong tissue especially at all joints throughout the body. It is the major tissue that hold bones together. When its injured its usually called a sprain or tear.

- Joint capsule: Similar to a ligament in that it helps hold two bones together to maintain a joint, but it is also very elastic, surrounds the joint and is filled with a type of fluid which helps keep the joint surface smooth and limit the friction. When its injured, its usually called a sprain or tear.

- Spinal cord: An extension of your brain which extends down the middle of your back bone and sends branches out through the small "hole" within the back bone to everywhere in your body. Messages about how things feel, how strong to contract a muscle, and balance are transmitted through the spinal cord.

How do I deal with a boss who needs to update equipment, but appears to be too cheap/frugal or unwilling to do so?

Some physical therapy facilities are more up to date than others, and have state of the art treatment and exercise equipment, while others do not. Working in a facility that has outdated equipment sometimes means that you as a therapist will be limited in your ability to perform certain interventions, and thus makes you less effective. This is a very frustrating thing when you are trying to establish your reputation as a new therapist. Before you go overboard by quitting the job and looking for another with up to date equipment, here are some suggestions to try first:

- Find a brochure of another clinic which has the same type of equipment you want your boss to purchase, and leave it sitting around in a very conspicuous place so that your boss can see it.

- Offer to donate some of your own salary. It's a low blow, and what's worse is that they may take you up on it. However, since you are a new graduate who is most certainly making the lowest salary possible and can't afford ant less money in your paycheck, there is a chance that the offer might make them feel guilty enough to make the investment.

- Show them how it contributes to decreased staff and patient morale, decreases staff retention, decreases facility reputation, increases cost, and thus decreases productivity.

- When a patient tells you that the lack of adequate exercise equipment at another clinic persuaded them to leave and come to your clinic, make sure your boss knows of this, so that the same thing won't happen to your clinic.

"If you want me to provide high level and safe physical therapy, this is the equipment that I will need from you". Adil Irani, MPT. Hagerstown, MD.

- Get a brochure from a competing physical therapy facility that offers the better equipment, and anonymously leave it on your supervisor's desk. Do this every day for as long as it takes for them to get the message. Just make sure that it's a really eye-popping brochure that shows the competing facility in a better light. Sometimes, a little competition makes the difference.

- Do a Google search for the websites of other facilities that offer the better equipment. Select the top ten websites that clearly are better due to possessing the better equipment, and then email the websites to your supervisor. Then ask them what they thought about idea. Sometimes visual presentation can paint a better picture in your supervisor's mind than your explanation can.

How do I deal with a patient who is also a medical professional, and who constantly attempts to challenge my knowledge and skills as a physical therapist?

Ok, here's the scene: you get an initial evaluation with a diagnosis of plantar fasciitis. You are made aware by the patient that she is a registered nurse, and that she works in subacute rehab facility. She constantly interrupts you as you speak. She questions the diagnosis of plantar fasciitis. She seems more interested in your educational background than she does with your plan of care. She repeatedly suggests other causes of the problem. When you go over the plan of care, she suggests other interventions. You try ultrasound, and she complains that she "doesn't feel anything" and suggests that you may have the wrong setting. You instruct her on therapeutic exercise, and she argues that she has a better way of performing them. Needless to say, this can be a very challenging, frustrating, and awkward situation. Here are some suggestions that may help guide you through this all too common scenario:

- Remember that although these scenarios are common, they are not always a problem. We as PT practitioners need to be challenged from time to time to keep us on our toes. So, every time the patient questions your decisions or changes the plan of care you have so carefully designed, don't get frustrated.

- Medical professionals challenge each other. Accept the challenges as learning experiences and motivation to learn the evidence. There's also tons of research that you can challenge their knowledge with their discipline.

- View it as a challenge that you must overcome by going beyond the call of duty, and providing the most unquestionably appropriate evaluation and intervention possible. Do extra research before every session with the patient.

- Read up and review the diagnosis even though you are already well-versed with the diagnosis. In this way, you will be ready for the challenge before it comes.

- Be honest. It's not a contest, so don't try to appear more clever and knowledgeable than they do.

- Remember that they came to you for help, and not the other way around.

- If you don't know or are unsure about anything the patient asks you, tell them what you DO know about it, and then inform them that you will let them know at the next session.

- Only state objective information and facts based on documented and researched evidence.

- Make sure you research and find out all there is to know before the next session, and then give them a heavy dose of the information.

- Take the position that you are there to help them, but if they believe they can treat themselves better, then you wish them well. (but don't say it) Say "I know you are a (medical doctor, nurse, occupational therapist, fireman, or whatever), and you may have seen different things, but I am just telling you what I've seen from MY OWN PERSONAL EXPERINCE.

How do I deal with a patient who is blind/deaf/mute/mentally handicap?

This is exactly the type of situation that will probably happen to you sooner or later, but most therapists were not specifically trained or prepared for this during school. This kind of situation can be very awkward if not handled properly, and the last thing you want as a therapist is to make your patient feel uncomfortable with you as their therapist. Here are some suggestions by others who have been in this situation before:

- If the patient is deaf make there is always a person who speaks sign language present

- If the patient is deaf, keep a notepad and pen available at all times in case you need to communicate by written word.

- If the patient is deaf, try to schedule treatments when family or friends are present so that they may be of assistance with communication.

- If the patient cannot speak, keep a pen and pad on hand.

- If the patient cannot speak, make sure you maintain eye contact with them because the patient's facial expression communicates a lot

- If the patient cannot speak, be sure not to leave the patient in a room unattended because if something negative should happen, there would be no way for you to know until it's too late.

- If the person is blind you must use touch as your communication aid. Manually guide the patient's body parts into the desired direction until they become independent with the motions.

- If the patient is blind, be sure to stay close with the patient at all times to avoids hazards such as falls, or other people colliding with the patient not knowing he/she was blind.

I need tips for dealing with a patient who speaks a different language?

There are times when a physical therapist will need to treat a patient who cannot answer pertinent health questions, has no clue of the meaning of the words that are spoken to him/her because the patient doesn't speak your language. This obviously makes for a very difficult physical therapy session for you as the therapist and for the person as the patient. Make no mistake about it, there will come a time when this will happen to you, and if you are reading this, it probably means it has already has, and you are looking for a way to handle it. Don't worry, help is on the way:

- Request that a family member or friend who speaks the patient's language and English be present at all times during the therapy session in order to translate.

- Prepare ahead of time by using the internet to find words and phrases that you will need to use at the next session.

- Download an app on your smart phone, and use it when speaking to the patient. Some apps even speak the words for you.

- Keep a translation reference book on hand when you know you will be seeing the patient who speaks another language, keep it in your back pocket or lab coat. Otherwise keep it on your desk or with the other reference texts at your job.

- Keep a pen and pad on hand for written communication if necessary. You will need to be creative by drawing figures or symbols such as pain scale.

- It is a good idea to find out if there are any staff members who actually knows how to speak the language in question, even if they are not fluent. This is actually the case more often than not, and especially when it comes to Spanish.

- Learn some of the most useful and highly used words and phrases such as "where does it hurt", "please stand up", or "pain".

How do I handle a situation where my patient has suffered a significant/severe setback in progress with physical therapy due to unknown reasons?

In most cases, physical therapy is a progress which occurs in stages, and is sometimes very difficult and hard work for the patient. The patient works hard because they know that it usually pays off with favorable results. However, sometimes, the progress that the patient was making suddenly reverses or slows down significantly, and there often appears to be no particular reason for it. These patients then often lose hope, become less compliant, and question your methods. This is obviously an awkward situation that no physical therapist wants to be in, especially if the therapist is a new grad. Never fear, we have all been there, and here are some of our suggestions:

- Explain to the patient that periodic setbacks in progress during physical therapy are very common and a normal and expected part of the rehabilitation process.

- Re-evaluate the patient, and determine if there is a specific reason for the setback. If there is, let the patient know that you will address it with a change in plan of care.

- Explain to the patient that periodic advanced improvements are also a normal part of the rehabilitation process, and advise them to look forward to them.

- Inform the patient that you do not expect the setback to remain for any extended period of time, and expect that he/she will bounce back just as suddenly as the setback came on.

- If it is in an outpatient setting where the patient comes to physical therapy several times a week, but lives at home, discuss what he/she is doing at home that may be causing this setback, especially things that they started doing near the time they initially noticed the setback. Whatever they were doing, recommend that they temporarily discontinue that activity and watch for an improvement in symptoms. If the setback reverses itself, then that activity was probably the culprit, so you must advise the patient to cease that activity while progressing through physical therapy.

How do I deal with a boss who has a policy of placing so many patients on my schedule, that I do not have enough time to properly treat them?

Don't worry, this is a common problem within physical therapy practice. Many staff physical therapists complain about having too many patients with too little time to treat them while ensuring a high level of quality. It could be due to the facilities regulations, and the boss has no say in the matter. It could be due to the boss desiring more profits as primary goal. It could be due to the boss not being aware that there are too many patients on your schedule. Despite the reason for it, the best thing to do is act on your feelings, because the worst thing you can do is remain silent and allow your quality of treatment to fall to an unacceptable level because you're afraid to talk to your boss. So here are some words of wisdom:

- Give them your two-week notice. You went to school for too long, and incurred too much debt to work like a horse.

- First, do your absolute best to make the situation work, and make sure that your boss takes notice of your efforts. Then, when things get unreasonably difficult and it all starts to unravel, go to your boss and explain the reason you must treat fewer patients per hour.

- Explain how scheduling practices are affecting quality of care

- Gather as many OBJECTIVE reasons why a decrease in your particular patient load would prove to be advantageous. Further, gather as many OBJECTIVE reasons why not initiating a decrease in your patient load would place the facility at a disadvantage.

  Examples of advantages for changing:
  -Decrease risk of costly mistakes
  -Gives more time to spend with the patient, who then gives positive feedback about the facility
  -Will make the patients happy enough to refer their friends and family
  -Improve quality
  -Helps provide more time to allow for proper documentation
  -Heavy load often lowers PT retention
  -Gives more time to learn to be more independent in the future

  Examples of disadvantages of not changing:
  -Employee morale stays low, and it shows
  -Not getting enough time to learn to become more efficient
  -You will remain concerned about possible liability issues
  -Inadequate supervision for Aides/Techs will continue to be a cause for poor performance.

- Talk to co-workers and find out what they think. Generally, if your co-workers don't think it's too much, it probably isn't. In that case, drop the idea of asking for a permanent change. Ask for a temporary decrease in patient load while you learn and work on becoming more efficient. Then work diligently on learning management strategies. You need to become more efficient fast.

How do I deal with a situation in which I am expected to treat a condition that I am simply not comfortable or confident in treating?

There are times when a patient may require or benefit from a specific technique or modality that you are not yet experienced in and therefore uncomfortable with performing. It's important to remember that it happens all the time, and its nothing to be ashamed of. In fact, recognizing that you're not yet ready to perform the treatment shows a higher level of maturity.

- Whatever you do, don't just "wing it" in order to avoid a sticky situation. The situation can get really sticky if something goes wrong while your "winging it", and it probably will.

- Chances are that if you're a new physical therapist, you do not have a lot of real-world experience, and your supervisor is fully aware of this. Talk with your supervisor. Explain your worries, and ask for their guidance and input. It will show that you are eager to do things right, and will also ease the supervisors mind of worrying if you are going to hurt a patient.

- Ask your supervisor if you can just assist another therapist while they perform the task for the first few times so that you may learn, and become comfortable performing the task independently. Let the supervisor know that after that, you will be more than happy to perform the task independently.

"Talk to your supervisor, and explain how overloading your schedule with patients negatively effects the practice".
Daniel Curtis, PT, DPT. Orlando, FL.

- Sit your supervisor down, and have an honest conversation with them. Your supervisor will understand if you are not quite comfortable with treating a particular condition as a new physical therapist. In fact, they will expect this situation to eventually occur, and they will be willing to either help guide you through the appropriate treatment, treat the patients themselves, or assign the patient to someone else until you become more experienced and comfortable.

- Do your research and educate yourself. If still not comfortable then refer to another clinician.

- If it is something you believe you SHOULD NOT be comfortable with, and no therapist should be doing, inform your supervisor of your feelings, and be firm in stating your case. If you have a good supervisor, he/she will look upon you favorably, and will then make the necessary arrangements to resolve the situation.

- If it is something that you SHOULD be comfortable with, don't immediately run to the supervisor. Take some initiative, and tell another therapist that this is your first time, and ask them to help walk you through the process the first (or second) time. Be sure to take good notes, and then do it independently the next time.

How do I deal with a patient in a situation where they were not appropriate for physical therapy even though they were referred to you by their doctor?

There are times when a physician is not sure of the patient's condition or how to treat it. If it even remotely appears to that a physical therapist maybe the discipline that is most appropriate for the patient, the physician will refer that patient to you. However, there are often times when, although physical therapy may seem like the appropriate intervention for the patient, it is not.

- After a thorough evaluation, inform the patient why they are not a candidate for physical therapy, inform the patient that you will inform his/her doctor of your findings, and suggest that they return to their referring doctor.

- Be sure to let your supervisor know of your decision not to treat the patient and ask for suggestions before you tell the patient, because as a new therapist, you could simply be wrong in your assessment.

- If you will not be treating the patient because of their inappropriateness for physical therapy, provide options such as referral to a specialist, home exercise instructions, general advice based on your professional judgement, or information on their condition such as general treatment options.

- Always perform a full evaluation of the patient's condition before making the decision that they are inappropriate for physical therapy. You might find something that validates their appropriateness for PT.

- Document objective data such as ROM, strength, balance, etc. Make note that they are within normal limits. Also document functional status such as ambulation, functional mobility, functional reach, etc. Then make note that all are within normal limits. Make the statement that "patient does not require physical therapy at this time".

How can I be sure that my plan of care is appropriate for the patient?

Confidence in your own skills and chosen treatment technique is very important because if you do not appear confident to the patient, the patient may lose confidence and trust in you as a competent physical therapist. When that happens, it will be very difficult to rebuild that crucial level of trust. Here are some suggestions on how to maintain confidence in your interventions:

- Go over your POC with another therapist (staff or otherwise)

- Compare your POC with textbook general treatment guidelines for the particular condition

- Review the plan of care with the patient, ask for any objections or concerns, and modify
- Accordingly

- If it is comparable to textbook interventions, rest assured that you're on the right track

- Ask the patient for their opinion of results periodically throughout therapy

How do I deal with another therapist who just can't seem to get along with me regardless of the reason, and who causes unnecessary problems for me?

- Schedule a meeting with the other physical therapist, and then have an honest discussion.

- Inform your supervisor of the situation, but let them know that you will be having a sit-down conversation with the other physical therapist in order to get down to the bottom of the problem and resolve it. But let your supervisor know that you may need to involve them if it doesn't go so well. If the conversation goes well and the situation is resolved, let your supervisor know that their assistance will not be necessary (trust me when I say that they will be grateful to you for making their life easier). But if it doesn't go well, then ask them for assistance.

- Discuss the situation with the other physical therapist after work over a beer

How do I deal with a situation where the patient is not improving with therapy?

Unfortunately, this scenario is a regular part of physical therapy. It does happen to patients for various reasons, and can be frustrating to the patient and physical therapist alike. This leads patient and therapist down an awful road of depression and doubt which can negatively affect the future outcome for both. The patient can lose confidence in the physical therapist, which can partly lead to the therapist losing confidence in him/herself, causing both to make unnecessary mistakes in a desperate struggle to see improvement.

- Consult with colleagues at your practice facility, fellow former classmates, and other physical therapists who are not at your practice facility.

- Be sure to inform the patient about any possible options they may have so that they are not left in the darkness about their future. This makes things easier for you and the patient. Even though the patient will not have made significant improvement, they patient will be grateful for your help because you have steered them toward the right direction in their journey toward improvement with their condition.

- Make sure to document all objective measurements along the way so that you can refer to objective measurements when discharging a patient

- Inform the patient that it is your professional opinion that they have probably reached a plateau in improvement and continued therapy will probably not improve their condition at this point.

- Inform the patient that since Pt does not seem to be helping much at this point, you will be referring him/her back to the physician who will probably run additional tests, and try other methods of treatment.

- Discharge the patient with three levels of individual exercises (beginning, intermediate, and advanced) which will allow the patient to progress him/herself from one level to the next independently.

- If you are discharging the patient be sure to give them your card with phone number on it, and remind them that they can call you with any questions about their condition if they cannot reach their doctor.

How do I contact my patient's doctor, voice a concern, and get results?

There are times when the therapist needs to contact the doctor and discuss tings related to a mutual patient for the benefit of that patient.

The therapist may need to ascertain any weightbearing restrictions or precautions, may need to clarify results from imaging, or may discuss something very important about the patient that the doctor may be unaware of. However, most doctors are very busy throughout the day, so they don't usually have a lot of time to spend on calls from therapists. If they are pulled away from performing their job and forced to talk to a person on the phone, there is a good chance that they may be irritated and short-tempered with the person on the other end of the phone. Add to this the fact that there are salespeople who routinely waste doctor's time by calling them on the phone, only to attempt a sale of some sort. Further, if you are timid and don't appear that you know what you're talking about, they may not take you seriously or even be angry with you for wasting their time. They don't like to be bothered all the time, especially by someone who appears to them as a physical therapist fresh from graduation who is over eager to impress them. If the doctor believes you will be bothering him/her every time they refer a patient to your facility, they may be less willing to do so, and this will not go over well with your supervisor or the director of your facility. How do you handle this tricky situation? Here are some really good suggestions that have worked well with other physical therapists:

To avoid making nervous mistakes, write down exactly what you want to discuss in bullet points before you make the call. and have it on hand as a script so that you won't forget anything and need to call back. Then check off each point as you discuss it with the doctor.

- Be very clear and to the point.

- Write down all of the pertinent information beforehand. Be short, brief, and straight to the point. That referring doctor usually doesn't have a lot of time to spend on the phone, and will appreciate your consideration.

- -Start the conversation off with your name, your title, who you work for, the name of the doctor's patient you are treating, and your reason for calling. Here is an example: "My name is John Doe, and I'm a physical therapist at Hands-On Physical Therapy and Athletic Rehabilitation Center. I am treating a patient by the name of John Doe whom you referred to us for treatment, and I am calling because I have a concern about this patient and I want to discuss it with you". This is helpful for many reasons. It immediately lets the doctor know that you're not a salesman. It says to the doctor that you're a colleague in the healthcare field. It tells the doctor that it's an important call because the health and wellness of his patient is at stake. It allows the doctor to realize that the call was ultimately a result of his action, so he will be inclined toward taking it more seriously. Most importantly, it allows the doctor to realize that you are actually doing him/her a favor, and if the doctor is a good doctor he/she is more eager to hear you out and thankful for your call.

- Since doctors see lots of patients every day, they may not instantly remember the patient you are referring to by name. Instead of simply mentioning the patient you are calling about, try to help jog the doctor's memory about which one of his many patients you are referring to by mentioning any unusual thing about the patient (for example: The tall gentleman who injured his knee when he slipped on ice).

- Be very professional, but friendly, and let the doctor know that if he/she has any concerns about any of the patients he/she refers to your office you welcome his/her call. This makes it easier to call that doctors office the next time you need to.

- Don't ask to talk with the doctor. Instead, leave a message for the doctor to call you at his/her earliest convenience regarding his/her patient.

How do I deal with a situation where a patient would benefit from continued therapy and would like to do so, their doctor also writes a script for continuation, but insurance won't allow?

This is a very common occurrence within physical therapy. Although, as a physical therapist in this situation you may feel hopeless, there actually are things you can do to either prevent this from happening, delay the inevitable, or even reverse the decision of the patient's insurance company. The following are all very good suggestions.

- First, make sure that your documentation supports continuation. This is done simply by showing objective measurements, which improve on a regular basis since the start of PT. The most observed and highly scrutinized objective measurements are ROM, strength, functional ability, gait, pain, and independence with HEP. Every time there is an improvement in these areas demonstrated through objective measurements, DOCUMENT IT in daily notes and especially in re-evaluations.

- Don't use the term script to start with. Offer patient self-pay option, but only after appealing with insurance company first. This way, the patient knows you have given them all of the available options, and they will be grateful to you for it.

- In addition to documenting objective measurements, you MUST actually STATE the need for continuation. This can also simply be incorporated into your regular daily notes and especially in re-evaluations. Use phrases such as the following: "Patient is making steady progress as seen with improved ROM, strength, and tolerance to therapeutic exercise. However, he has not yet reached full potential from PT and should benefit from continued PT in order to address remaining unmet goals established during initial evaluation". Other examples are "Pt is making slow, but steady progress toward established goals", "Pt's recent improvement in ROM is showing increased potential for overall improvement, provided he continues with current POC, and "Although pt had a mild setback in progress due to pain, now that pain is subsiding, he is now able to tolerate manual therapy and therapeutic exercises much better. This should drastically increase his potential for improvement".

- Write up a generic note which you can later insert individual names and specific information about a patient who has been denied continuation of therapy by his/her health insurance. Keep the generic note filed onto a computer to be used when needed. The note must include the following things:
Clearly state why therapy continuation is necessary
Clearly state why you believe the patient has good potential for improvement (must be objective)
Clearly demonstrate that objective measurements are improving on a steady basis
Clearly state the reason the patient was not showing improvement, and also show that the reason has now been resolved.

Clearly note that changes in POC will take place in response to the patient's new status, now that the reason for lack of improvement has been resolved.

- If all else fails, consult with the patient and make him/her aware of the situation. Be completely honest. Let the patient know that you recommend more therapy, and their doctor agrees, but the insurance company won't budge. Instruct the patient with several progressive levels of home exercises so they can progress to the higher levels as they improve at home. Give the patient a business card (if your facility supplies one for you), and make sure they understands that if they have any questions or concerns, they can contact you personally. In this way, the patient is comfortable knowing that you are in their corner and did everything in your power to help them improve. Talk about respect for you as a physical therapist, this patient may go home, cancel their health insurance, obtain another type, and personally call your facility asking to be treated by you and only you. Ok, that may be an exaggeration, but your supervisor will take note of your competence, which promotes great job security, and you will get a big boost in confidence knowing that you did handled a very uncomfortable and potentially volatile situation in outstanding fashion.

- If you are really feeling particularly lucky, contact the insurance company, and with the patient's chart in hand, ask for the representative's name and then ask the representative to explain the denial decision. If the decision was based on lack of patient improvement, outline the objective measurements and point out specific areas of improvement. If the decision was based on limitations in the patient's policy such as a cap in benefits, ask the representative if there are any exemptions or exceptions based on special circumstances, and what steps you need to take in order to qualify for these exceptions. Sometimes, denials are due to missing documentation or illegible handwriting. Sometimes, it is simply a matter of re-faxing a particular document. The key is to find the specific reason for denial and try to correct it.

- Call the insurance company and obtain a contact name in reference to the patients claim. After explaining the situation to the patient, and informing him/her that you have already attempted to contact the insurance company in order to request additional visits and was unsuccessful, give them the telephone number and name of the person you talked with. Tell the patient to give them a call because there are some times when insurance companies will be more reasonable when requests for more approval for more treatment is coming from more than one source.

- If it's near the end of the calendar year, and the denial is because the patient has reached the maximum amount of treatment per their particular insurance plan, I sometimes explain that fact to the patient, and instruct them on enough home exercises to get them through to the new year. This is because the insurance benefits usually start fresh at that point, and the patient will be allowed more visits. I tell the patient to come back again if they feel the need to do so after January 1st.

Useful everyday phrases:

There are some ideas that we as physical therapists try to communicate to our patients every day in order to help them understand or remember this very important information. It's a good idea to develop some of your own, but here are some that may be useful to you in your practice.

- An answer to the question how do you know how far to stretch is "come as close as you can to the door of pain but don't walk through it".

- "On a scale of one to ten, how much pain do you experience on average. Zero is no pain, ten is passing out from pain".

- "The rehab process is like charting a progress on a graph. There are hills and valleys along the way, but as long as you have more hills than valleys on your way to the top you're ok".

- "How did the home exercises go?".

- "Make a mental note about how you feel after performing these home exercises, and let me know at your next session because the exercises that you will be performing in the clinic will be partially dependent on how you do with the home exercises".

- "This is sort of the trial period. We want to see what level of exercise your body will and will not tolerate, so we will start off very light and progress from there."

- In an outpatient setting and after the completion of the patient's session, in order to help prevent no-shows due to forgetting the next appointment, its sometimes helpful to say "see you in a couple days…wait…what is it, (and then just throw any day in there) Wednesday?" If they don't correct you or tell you for sure when their appointment is, tell them to check with the receptionist on the way out.

- "Watch your step. No falling allowed around here".

- "When it appears that the patient is holding their breath against your advice you can say "your turning red again".

Suggested acronym for remembering carpal bones:

As a physical therapist, you will be working with patient's injured wrists, so it's obviously important for you to remember the names and positions of each carpal bone, but any PT will tell you that for whatever reason, it's not as easy as it may seem. For this reason, physical therapists have supplemented their memory with the use of acronyms. Here are some acronyms that are often used by veteran physical therapists, hope it helps.

- Some Lovers Tried Positions That They Couldn't Handle

- Sally Left Tom Pushing The Third Cart Home

- Stay Low To Pop The Top Cop Hop

- Suzy Let The Pet Try To Catch Her

- She Looks Too Pretty, Try To Catch Her

- P T's Love Sex However Can't Take Time

- Send Lilly To Paris To Tame Carnal Hunger

Suggested acronym for remembering tarsal bones:

As a physical therapist, it goes without saying that you will encounter patients with conditions of the foot involving the tarsal bones. Unfortunately, as with the carpal bones, it is extremely difficult to remember and differentiate the names, positions, and functions of each of the many tarsal bones after you graduate your physical therapy program of study and begin concentrating on the one hundred thousand other things required of you as a newly practicing physical therapist. Remembering the names and positions of each tarsal bones is tremendously effective in eliciting recollection of everything else about the tarsal bones. This is the reason it is important to have a system that allows you to recall the tarsal bones on demand when you encounter that patient with the foot condition. Here are some suggestions.

- The Cab in New Mexico Is Land Cruiser

- The Cure of Nemaline Myopathy Is of Least Concern

- Tall Californian Navy Medical Interns Lay Cuties

- Tiger Cub Needs MILC

Suggested acronym for remembering cranial nerves and functions:

Ahh, those hard to remember cranial nerves. You know you need to know them, but how is it humanly possible to remember them all. Well, my colleague, you have just struck gold!!! Here are some acronyms that may prove very helpful. Repeat any of them in a self-composed melody, and you will remember them forever.

- Oliver the Optimistic Octopus Trots Triumphantly About Facing Audiences Glossily Vaguely Spinning Hippos. (Note that the accessory nerve is referred to by its alternate name Spinal accessory nerve, and the Vestibulocochlear nerve by its former name, Auditory, in this mnemonic.)

- On Old Olympus' Towering Top A Fin And German Viewed Some Hops. (Note that the accessory nerve is referred to by its alternate name Spinal accessory nerve, and the Vestibulocochlear nerve by its former name, Auditory, in this mnemonic.).

- Ooh, Ooh, Ooh To Touch And Feel Very Good Velvet. Such Heaven! (Note that the accessory nerve is referred to by its alternate name Spinal accessory nerve in this mnemonic.)

- Oh Once One Takes The Anatomy Final Very Good Vacations Are Heavenly. And to help remember the types of information these nerves carry (sensory, motor, or both) use: Some Say Marry Money, But My Brother Says Big Brains Matter More.

Dermatome memorization tricks:

Dermatomes can sometimes be tricky to remember, especially if your not working in a neuro setting or rarely see patients with neurological conditions. However, regardless of the practice setting, you will eventually need to assess dermatomes. So, it is in your best interest to have a system that, regardless of how long it's been since you have needed to asses them, allows you to recall the dermatome patterns on demand. Here are some suggestions.

- Whenever you perform an initial evaluation, it is always helpful to have a clipboard with a dermatome diagram printed on the front surface of the clipboard for easy, reference. You can purchase these clipboards from any book store which sells medical texts. You can also make a copy of a dermatome chart from a textbook and tape it to your clipboard for easy reference.

- ✓ Dermatome sites:
- ✓ C2 at Occipital protuberance

- ✓ C3 just above the clavicle
- ✓ C4 near AC joint
- ✓ C5 near lateral antecubital fossa
- ✓ C6 at the thumb.
- ✓ C7 anterior index finger
- ✓ C8 Middle finger
- ✓ T1 Near medial antecubital fossa
- ✓ T2 Within the armpit
- ✓ T3-T12 descending from upper to lower anterior trunk
- ✓ T4 at the nipple.
- ✓ T10 at the umbilicus.L1 Upper anterior thigh
- ✓ L2 Mid anterior thigh (The middle of the quad is where it runs through)
- ✓ L3 Medial femoral condyle (what else can it be but inside the knee)
- ✓ L4 Medial Malleolus (the bump on the inside of the ankle contour)
- ✓ L5 Near dorsum of big toe (if you trip over it you take a dive)S1 Near lateral heel (stepping on a tack can be no fun)
- ✓ S2 Near Popliteal fossa (behind the knee can be black and blue)
- ✓ S3 - S4 at the perineum. (all at the back door)

Myotome memorization tricks:

Knowing and understanding Myotomes is obviously a vital part of our practice, and it is well understood that every physical therapist should know them. However, our brains are not computers that store everything in a hard drive forever as long as coffee is not spilled onto it. We are humans. We forget!!! Learn the following phrases, and other therapists will think your brain really is a computer. Here is a little help:

- ✓ "C3 4 and 5 diaphragm breathing to keep me alive"

- ✓ C5 also supplies the shoulder muscles and the muscle that we use to bend our elbow .

- ✓ "C5 alone make a muscle, move your shoulder bone

- ✓ C6 flicks the wrist.

- ✓ C7 keeps the elbows straight like to heaven

- ✓ "C8- Don't wait, squeeze my hand and don't hesitate"

- ✓ "T1 makes it fun to spread your fingers like bubble gum

- ✓ T1 –T12ish chest and abs can be selfish.

- ✓ L2 flexes the hip like no other will do

- ✓ L3 kicks the knee like Bruce Lee

- ✓ L4 keeps your toes from hitting the flo (floor)

- ✓ L5 wiggles toes that are five. My feet are alive

- ✓ S1 "it. Plant your feet down and gun it..

- ✓ S3 through five makes pelvic muscles thrive.

Good lumbosacral plexus acronyms

The lumbosacral Plexus, an extremely complicated web of specific nerves that are vital to lower extremities. Yet, it is nearly impossible to remember the organization of these nerves. If only there was a method of visualizing the organization of these nerves in your mind, you would be a better physical therapist. Well, have no fear, veteran physical therapists are here! The following are examples of methods to remember the organization of the lumbosacral Plexus.

- "**I, I G**et **L**aid **O**n **F**ridays":
  Iliohypogastric [L1]
  Ilioinguinal [L1]
  Genitofemoral [L1, L2]
  Lateral femoral cutaneous [L2, L3]
  Obturator [L2, L3, L4]
  Femoral [L2, L3, L4]

- "**I** twice **G**et **L**aid **O**n **F**ridays".

- "Interested In Getting Laid On Fridays?

- **"2 from 1, 2 from 2, 2 from 3"**:
  2 nerves from **1** root: Ilioinguinal (L1), Iliohypogastric (L1).
  2 nerves from **2** roots: Genitofemoral (L1,L2), Lateral Femoral (L2,L3).
  2 nerves from **3** roots: Obturator (L2,L3,L4), Femoral (L2,L3,L4).

- **"MAP OF Sciatic"**:
  Medial compartment: **O**bturator
  Anterior compartment: **F**emoral
  Posterior compartment:
  Sciatic: So all the thigh muscles in that compartment get innervated by that nerve.

DTR acronym

As with dermatomes, myotomes, cervical plexus, etc. Memorizing all of the Deep Tendon Reflexes and their corresponding nerve roots is difficult, especially if you work in a practice setting where conditions seen do not typically require assessment of deep tendon reflexes. Its similar to what happens when you can speak a second language, but slowly forget words and phrases within that language because you don't live in an area where the people speak that language. You can bet that you will eventually run into a person who speak that language, and you don't want to struggle to remember the words when speaking to that person. Similarly, regardless of the practice setting, there will still be times when you need to assess deep tendon reflexes, and you don't want to find yourself drawing a blank when it's time to assess them. Here are some suggested acronyms to help you recall all of the DTRs on demand.

- **"1,2,3,4,5,6,7,8"**:
  S**1-2**: ankle
  L**3-4**: knee
  C**5-6**: biceps, supinator
  C**7-8**: triceps
  One, two..buckle my shoe. **Three, four**..kick the door. **Five, six**..pick up sticks. **Seven, eight**..shut the gate.

- **S1,2** = ankle jerk
- **L3,4** = knee jerk
- **C5,6** = biceps and brachioradialis
- **C7,8** = triceps

How do I memorize the Brachial Plexus once and for all?

In order to perform a good evaluation of upper extremity neurologic disfunction, you should obviously be able to differentiate between the nerve origins, which means you need to know the brachial plexus like the back of your hand. Unfortunately, memorizing the brachial plexus is an extremely difficult task. That is unless you utilize some of the following acronyms suggested by other physical therapists.

- It is the same backwards and forwards:
  5-3-2-3-5:
  5 Rami
  3 Trunks
  2 Divisions
  3 Cords
  5 Terminal nerves

- **STAR:**
  Subscapular [upper and lower]
  Thoracodorsal
  Axillary
  Radial

- "**R**andy **T**ravis **D**rinks **C**old **B**eer":
  Roots
  Trunks
  Divisions
  Cords
  Branches

- "**R**ead **T**he **D**amn **C**adaver **B**ook!"

- "**R**eal **T**exans **D**rink **C**oors **B**eer".

- "**T**he **C**astrated **D**og **T**urns **R**abid" (From lateral to medial):

111

Terminal branches
Cords
Divisions
Trunks
Roots

- "My Aunt Raped My Uncle" (From lateral to medial):
Musculocutaneous
Axillary
Radial
Median
Ulnar

- "Robert Tried Drinking Cold Beer"

Which medications and their effects do you think a therapist should know and understand?

As a physical therapist, there will be times when your treatment options will be limited by the medications that your patient is currently taking. For instance, if your patient has a history of heart problems, and is currently taking heart medications, so your plan is to monitor their heart rate while they ride the stationary bike, you may not be able to monitor their heart rate because the medications may be designed to prevent their heart rate from increasing, regardless of the intensity of the exercise. Its best to know the name of this medication so that you can modify your plan accordingly. Another example is if your patient suddenly complains of dizziness during exercise, if you know that dizziness is a side-effect of the medications they are currently taking, you can make better decisions in how you handle the situation. Here are some of the more common medications that your patients take which may affect your interventions.

- Name: Dobutamine HCL
Generic: Dobutrex
Use: Heart condition
Adverse effects: Headache, nausea, increased systolic BP, increased HR, palpitations, angina

- Name: Dopamine
Generic: Inotropin

112

Use: Heart condition
Adverse effects: Nausea, vomiting, tachycardia, angina pain, dyspnea, hypotension, palpitations

- Name: Levalbuterol
  Generic: Xopenex
  Use: bronchialspasm
  PT related side effects: nausea, sweating, pallor, flushing

- Name: Acebutalol HCL
  Generic: Sectral
  Use: Hypertension, arrhythmia
  Side affects relevant to PT: Bradycardia, dizziness, weakness, hypotension, nausea, vomiting.

- Name: Atenolol
  Generic: Tenormin
  Use: Hypertension, arrhythmia
  Adverse effects: Bradycardia, dizziness, weakness, hypotension, nausea, vomiting, fatigue

- Name: Betaxolol
  Generic: Kerlone
  Use: Hypertension
  Side effects relevant to PT: Bradycardia, dizziness, hypotension, bronchospasm, nausea, vomiting.

- Name: Bisopolol
  Generic: Zebeta
  Use: Hypertension
  Side affects relevant to PT: Bradycardia, dizziness, weakness, hypotension, nausea, vomiting

- Name: Carteolol
  Generic: cartrol
  Use: Hypertension
  Side affects relevant to PT: Bradycardia, hypotension, weakness, dizziness, vomiting

- Name: Penbutolol
  Generic: Levatol
  Use: Hypertension

Side affects relevant to PT: Bradycardia, dizziness, hypotension, nausea, vomiting.

- Name: carvedilol
  Generic: Coreg
  Use: Hypertension, CHF
  Side affects relevant to PT: Bradycardia, hypotension, fatigue, dizziness.

- Name: Labetalol
  Generic: Normodyne/Trandate
  Use: Hypertension
  Side affects relevant to PT: Tafigue, Drowsiness, hypotension

- Name: Prazosin
  Generic: Minipress
  Use: Hypertension
  Side affects relevant to PT: Dizziness, postural hypotension, drowsiness, strength loss, palpitations,
  Headache

- Name: Terazosin
  Generic: Hytrin
  Use: Hypertension, BPH
  Side affects relevant to PT: Postural hypotension, dizziness, dyspnea, headache.

- Name: Phenilzine
  Generic: Nardil
  Use: Depression
  Side affects relevant to PT: Orthostatic hypotension, dizziness, nausea, and blurred vision

- Name: Trancylcypromine
  Generic: Parnate
  Use: Depression
  Side affects relevant to PT: Orthostatic hypotension, dizziness, nausea, and blurred vision

- Name: Citalopram
  Generic: Celexia
  Use: Depression

Side affects relevant to PT: Orthostatic hypotension, dizziness, nausea, tremor

- Name: Fluoxetine
  Generic: Prozac, Sarafem
  Use: Depression
  Side affects relevant to PT: fatigue, dizziness, nausea.

- Name: Sertraline
  Generic: Zoloft
  Use: Depression, OCD, PTSD
  Side affects relevant to PT: Fatigue, dizziness.

- Name: Venlafaxine
  Generic: Effexor
  Use: Depression, anxiety disorder
  Side affects relevant to PT: Dizziness, paresthesia, weakness.

- Name: Phenytoin Sodium
  Generic: Dilantin
  Use: Epilepticus, seizures
  Side affects relevant to PT: Ataxia, Nystagmus, dizziness, mental confusion.

- Name: Entacapone
  Generic: Comtan
  Use: Parkinson's Disease
  Side affects relevant to PT: Orthostatic hypotension, dyskinesia, dystonia, dizziness, nausea, muscle cramps.

- Name: Fentanyl
  Generic: Sublimaze
  Use: Analgesic
  Side affects relevant to PT: Sedation, vertigo, lethargy, nausea

- Name: Oxycodone
  Generic: OxyContin
  Use: Analgesic
  Side affects relevant to PT: Light-headedness, sedation, dizziness, nausea.

- Name: Propoxyphene
  Generic: Darvocet, Darvon
  Use: Analgesic
  Side affects relevant to PT: Light-headedness, sedation, dizziness, nausea.

- Name: Loratadine
  Generic: Claratin, Claratitia
  Use: Allergic Rhinitis
  Side affects relevant to PT: Dizziness, tremors, blurred vision.

- -Vicodin
- -Skelaxin
- -Flexeril
- -Blood pressure meds
- -Blood thinner meds
- -Anti-depressant meds

- Name: Digoxin
  Generic: Digitex, Lanoxicaps, Lanoxin
  Use: Heart Failure and fibrillations
  Side affects relevant to PT: Weakness, drowsiness, nausea, visual disturbances

- Name: Nmlodipine
  Generic: Norvasc
  Use: HTN
  Side affects relevant to PT: Dizziness, nausea, peripheral edema, bradycardia

- Name: Verapamil
  Generic: Calan, Isoptin, Verelan
  Use: Essential HTN, angina
  Side affects relevant to PT: Dizziness, nausea, peripheral edema, bradycardia

- Name: Sectral
  Generic: Acebutolol HCL
  Use: HTN, arrhythmia
  Side affects relevant to PT: fatigue, Hypotension, weakness, bradycardia

- Name: Tenormin

Generic: Atenolol
Use: HTN, Angina
Side affects relevant to PT: Fatigue, Hypotension, weakness, bradycardia, blurred vision

- Name: Coreg
Generic: Carvedilol
Use: HTN, CHF
Side affects relevant to PT: Fatigue, orthostatic Hypotension, weakness, bradycardia

- Name: Trandate, Normodyne
Generic: Labetalol HCL
Use: HTN
Side affects relevant to PT: Fatigue, Orthostatic Hypotension, weakness, bradycardia

- Name: Toprol XL, Lopressor
Generic: Metoprolol
Use: HTN, Angina
Side affects relevant to PT: Fatigue, Hypotension, weakness, bradycardia

- Name: Vasotec
Generic: enalopril
Use: HTN
Side affects relevant to PT: Fatigue, headache, nausea

- Name: Coumadin
Generic: Warfarin
Use: venous thrombosis
Side affects relevant to PT: Hemorrhage

"Excessive bruising all on all parts of the body is much more likely to be a side effect of taking coumadin

medication than a sign of physical abuse". Mikhail Muhammad, BS, MPT, DPT, OCS, CSCS, SCS, CPT, Farmington Hills, MI

- Name: Heparin
  Generic: Heparin
  Use: venous thrombosis
  Side affects relevant to PT: Hemorrhage, bruising, hematoma

- Name: Lovenox
  Generic: Enoxaparin
  Use: DVT prophylaxis
  Side affects relevant to PT: Hemorrhage, bruising

- Name: Innohep
- Generic: Tinzaparin sodium
  Use: DVT
  Side affects relevant to PT: Hemorrhage, bruising, hypersensitivity, fever

- Name: Naturetin (a thiazide)
  Generic: Benzoflumethiazide
  Use: Edema due to CHF, HTN
  Side affects relevant to PT: Hypotension, dizziness, vertigo, nausea, weakness

- Name: Fosamax
  Generic: Alendronate sodium
  Use: Osteoporosis, Paget's disease
  Side affects relevant to PT: Recurrent bone pain, arthralgia, HA, nausea

- Name: Actonel
  Generic: Risedronate sodium
  Use: Osteoporosis, Paget's disease
  Side affects relevant to PT: Recurrent bone pain, arthralgia, HA, nausea

- Name: Flexeril

Generic: Cyclobenzaprine Hydrochloride
Use: Acute musculoskeletal pain and discomfort
Side affects relevant to PT: Drowsiness, dizziness, nausea

- Name: Soma
  Generic: carisoprodol
  Use: Acute musculoskeletal pain and discomfort
  Side affects relevant to PT: Drowsiness, dizziness, nausea, tachycardia

- Name: Dantrium
  Generic: Dantrolene Sodium
  Use: spasticity due to SCI, CVA, CP, or MS
  Side affects relevant to PT: Drowsiness, dizziness, weakness, malaise tachycardia

- Name: Valium
  Generic: Diazepam
  Use: Muscle spasticity due to CP, epilepsy, anxiety, or paraplegia
  Side affects relevant to PT: Drowsiness, sleepiness, sedation, lethargy, bradycardia, tachycardia

- Name: Roboxin
  Generic: Methocarbamol
  Use: Discomfort due to musculoskeletal disorders
  Side affects relevant to PT: Drowsiness, confusion, headache

- Name: Synvisc
  Generic: Hyaluronic acid
  Use: OA knee pain with no response to other treatment
  Side affects relevant to PT: swelling in involved knee, temporary pain, nausea, rash

The most frequently used and convenient special tests.

As a physical therapist, you have access to so many orthopedic special tests that it is sometimes difficult to decide on one to use. Some are faster and easier to perform, and thus help you improve your efficiency as a physical therapist. Some are better predictors of the source of the patient's problem. Some are less uncomfortable for the patient to undergo. Some are more appropriate for a given condition than another. And some can even be used to detect multiple conditions, which may make them a better test to use than a test that only helps to rule in or out one condition. No matter the reason, after researching which special tests have the highest validity and reliability, it is a good idea to have certain "go to" tests for a given body part. The following are some special tests that most often used by veteran physical therapists for this reason.

- **Cervical:**
  ✓ Spurlings test
  ✓ Upper Limb Tension tests
  ✓ Vertebral Artery Occlusion test
  ✓ Quadrant test
  ✓ Distraction test

- **Lumbar:**
  ✓ Quadrant test
  ✓ SI joint gapping test
  ✓ SI joint approximation test
  ✓ Tripod test
  ✓ SLR test
  ✓ Slump test

- **Shoulder:**
  ✓ Speed's test
  ✓ Ludington's test
  ✓ Drop-Arm test
  ✓ Neer's Impingement test
  ✓ Painful Arc test
  ✓ Anterior Apprehension test
  ✓ Cross-Arm Adduction Test
  ✓ AC Joint Shear test
  ✓ Yergason's test
  ✓ Empty Can test
  ✓ Hawkin's impingement test

- **Elbow:**
  ✓ Test for Lateral Epicondylitis
  ✓ Test for medial Epicondylitis
  ✓ Valgus Stret test
  ✓ Varus Stress test
  ✓ Elbow Flex test for Cubital Tunnel Syndrome

✓ Test for Pronator teres Syndrome

- **Wrist/Hand:**
✓ Finkelsteins test
✓ Phalen's test
✓ Froment's Sign
✓ Pinch test
✓ Wartenberg's sign
✓ Tinels sign

- **Hip:**
✓ Thomas's test
✓ Ober's test
✓ Sign of Buttock test
✓ Faber's test
✓ Trendelenberg test
✓ SLR test
✓ Scouring test
✓ Obers test

- **Knee:**
✓ Anterior Drawer test
✓ Lachman's test
✓ Pivot-Shift test
✓ Apley's Grinding test
✓ Clarke's sign
✓ Posterior drawer test
✓ McMurrey's test
✓ Noble's Compression test
✓ Valgus stress test
✓ Varus stress test
✓ Patella Apprehension test

- **Ankle/foot:**
✓ Anterior Drawer test
✓ Single Leg Heel Raise
✓ Talar Tilt test
✓ Kleiger's test
✓ Squeeze test
✓ Homan's signThompson's test
✓ Metatarsal Loading test
✓ Morton's neuroma test

How do I deal with a situation where my patient makes it known that they want to be seen by another therapist instead of me because I am new or seem too young, and so they don't trust my opinion?

Have you ever boarded a plane and happen to catch a glimpse of the pilot who seemed really young to be a commercial airline pilot, and felt that he may not have enough experience to fly the plane as safe as a veteran pilot? Of course, you have, and its only human nature. But unlike airline pilots, you don't have the luxury of making them just strap in and have faith in your skill level. Your patients have the option to simply refuse to be seen by you or even walk out, so you actually need to make sure the patient is comfortable in your skills as a physical therapist. How in the world are you supposed to do this? Strap in and have faith in your colleagues who are veteran physical therapist. They have some pretty good suggestions.

- Be honest and straightforward in letting them know that you are noticing the hesitance or resistance to your help and wonder if it is because you appear young or inexperienced. Allow them to acknowledge the fact. Then explain how selective and competitive the PT program is, and give a brief synopsis of your education, and how rigorous your training was. Then reassure the patient that they are in good hands.

- Tell them that you understand, and then allow them to see another physical therapist. It may not be worth attempting to overcome the patient's preconceived bias. Furthermore, it may not even be possible.

- Don't take it personal because it is not personal. Understand that the patient simply is unaware of your skill level, and wants to be reassured that he/she is receiving competent treatment. Put yourself in the patient's shoes, and you may feel the same way, so be very understanding when you reply.

- Immediately stop treatment, bring the patient in a private non-threatening area, and sit them down for a one-on-one conversation. Tell them that you sense something wrong with them, and would like to know what it is. Tell them that they can be perfectly honest with you. Gently rub their shoulder, sit close to them, look deeply into their eyes, whatever it takes, but just get them to confess. When they do confess, show that you are relieved. Tell them that this has happened before (if it has), but that after the initial concern wore off, the patient made excellent improvement. Let them know that there is nothing wrong with feeling that way. Explain to them that you are not upset or very surprised because you realize that you look young and inexperienced, but reassure them that once they get to know you through therapy sessions, they will realize just how good you really are.

- Tell the patient where you got your undergraduate degree from. Tell them where you got your graduate degree from. Then explain how rigorous the PT program of study is, and insure them that they are in good and qualified hands. You may be surprised that this is all the patient needed to be comfortable with you.

How do I deal with a lead therapist or supervisor who refuses to consider my suggestions because I am a new therapist or seem too young?

New physical therapists are not the only people who find themselves in this frustrating situation. This is a scenario that can play itself out in any profession. It can cause friction in the workplace, and make your workday uncomfortable and unhappy, and unnecessarily decrease how much you look forward to coming to work as the great physical therapist that you are. Before you embark on you quest to resolve this dreadful situation on your own, arm yourself with some of your PT colleagues suggested methods on dealing with situation. The following should be very helpful.
Those suggestions are as follows.

- Go over your suggestions with another staff therapist who has much more experience in the field than you, and get their opinion. If they like it, try to convince them to relay your suggestions to the supervisor.

- Obtain tangible evidence such as brochures from other facilities, magazines articles, or internet websites which demonstrate standards of practice that correlate to your suggestions.

- Write down as many reasons why your suggestions can benefit the facility financially, and bring the list to your supervisor.

- Document any instance where a patient's complaints could have been prevented by implementation of your suggestions, and re-submit the suggestions to your supervisor.

- Request a sit-down meeting with the supervisor or lead therapist, and honestly tell them your concerns. They may not even be aware that they are dismissing you, and will immediately begin to consider your suggestions.

- Ask the supervisor to give you their reasons for dismissing your suggestions. It could be that they simply have a better rationale than yours, and they have incorporated factors that you just didn't think of. But if this is not the case, this is the perfect opportunity to point out the reasons that your rationale is better, and that your suggestions should be implemented.

How do I deal with another therapist whose unprofessional or incompetent behavior is placing patients at risk and making me appear just as incompetent due to association?

This scenario is not one that occurs a lot in our profession because incompetent and unprofessional behavior is widely unacceptable among physical therapist colleagues. However, I included this scenario in this book because in the rare chance that this does occur, not only can it be very difficult to navigate through, but if not addressed appropriately, it can lead to a decrease in our standard of professionalism as physical therapists, and that is something that we cannot allow. Not to put a lot of pressure on you, it is very important that you handle this situation well. Thanks to your veteran PT colleagues, there is help. Read on.

- Do not associate with that therapist whatsoever, they are a cancer to our profession.

- Talk to the therapist, and ask them if you can be frank with them. Tell them that what they are doingis spilling out onto you and making it seem as though you are doing it.

- Tell them that you don't do that sort of thing, and don't want people to think that you do. Ask them to either stop doing what they are doing, or make sure that it doesn't appear that you had anything to do with it.

- If you have talked to them about it, and the problem continues, tell them that you are very concerned and upset about it because it is affecting your career, and not to take it personal but will give them another chance before you inform your supervisors.

- If the problem has not resolved after discussing it with the therapist twice, go to your supervisors. Tell them that you have already discussed it with the therapist twice privately, and you are not attempting to get them into trouble, but your integrity as a competent therapist is at stake, and you take that very seriously. Only after you have stated this do you inform them of the specific problem.

"Remind the therapist in private of what they are doing, because it is possible that they were simply unaware". Alex Pandya, MPT.

Rochester, MI

- Whatever you do, don't do what they are doing, and make it well known that you don't.

How do I deal with another therapist or health professional whom I work with on a daily basis, seeing the same patients, but who does not consult with you concerning important matters about the patients or does not coordinate their treatment with mine.

Nothing is worse than doing a chart review on a current patient whom you have never treated before, going into a room, initiating treatment per the plan of care in the patients chart, and the patient says "we don't do that anymore". Or even worse, initiating a plan of care for a patient, and another therapist completely disregarding your POC without documenting any changes. So, the next time you see the patient, it looks like you don't know what you're doing. It's enough to make you pull your hair out. Well don't go bald, trying to tackle this problem, here is help:

- Go to them and initiate discussion on a patient that you both treat. Ask them what they think about a particular patient that you both treat. Tell them your thoughts on that patient, especially useful things that they may have missed. Compare and contrast notes, so that they may see benefit in coordinating treatment.

- Inform the other therapist that you noticed that they changed your plan of care, and that you assume that they recognized a better course of action. Ask them to help you understand the rationale behind the new plan of care so that you can incorporate it into your practice next time. If they have no rationale, explain your rationale, and then inform them that it makes more sense to proceed with your original plan of care.

- Have a discussion with them and how their failure to consult is negatively impacting patient care

- If you are required to coordinate treatments between other health professionals such as nursing or OT, remind the other health professional. If you are new to the facility or a new therapist, tell them so. And tell them that it would make your life and job a whole lot easier if they would simply do their part. Everyone wants to help the "new guy", and this is an opportunity for them to do so.

- After reviewing the patient's POC, and before actually treating the patient, go to the previous therapist who is usually the source of the problem, and confirm with them that the documented POC and treatment intervention is still current. If they say no, inform them that you would like to continue sticking with the plan of care that was specifically devised for the patient's benefit, and that you will not be treating the patient without it (be firm on this). Then have them correct it immediately so that you can treat the patient properly. Then, and only then should you treat the patient. If this is done a few times, which would be just enough to bother that therapist enough to do it right the first time in order to avoid hearing from that pesky new physical therapist. Be careful, though, it may also embarrass the therapist because a new physical therapist needed to remind him/her to perform the job more competently, and you don't want to embarrass the people you work with (although it may be necessary in order to wake them up and make them do things properly).

How do I deal with another therapist who constantly points out my errors and faults in the open and in front of patients and colleagues?

Just like any other occupation, physical therapists all have their own personalities, and sometimes two of them can they collide with each other and cause friction. The important thing to remember is that it's not the end of the world. The answer is sometimes easier than you might think. Here are some suggestions.

- Wait until the two of you are in private, and let them know that you have noticed this, and it is really bothering you. If you are new, don't be ashamed. Instead, tell them that you are relatively new, and you are already trying to prove yourself, but pointing out your mistakes and highlighting your flaws are not helping. Tell them that they can help you become a better therapist by informing you of your errors and mistakes in private, and then adding some advice.

- While in public, don't show that it upsets you. Don't even discuss the fact that it is inappropriate to point out your flaws in public. This will only serve to make the problem bigger than it already is.

- Talk to their supervisor, only after attempting to work out the problem privately between yourself and the other person at least twice. Be sure to address any apparent mistakes that you have made before you go to your supervisor.

- Privately remind the person that it is unprofessional to point out your flaws and errors in public. But also let them know that you are very open to their suggestions in private. If they are a veteran therapist, they should realize that you did the right thing by pulling them aside in private, while they did the wrong thing by doing it public. They should get the message, and return the favor next time.

- As soon as it happens, give them a very stern facial expression without allowing the patient to see. Make sure that the expression grabs the other therapist's attention in such a manner that they will remember it later. After you have completed your therapy session with the patient, and you and the other therapist are alone. Ask them if they remember the expression you gave them. Tell them that you did that because you knew it would be inappropriate to discuss your disagreement in front of the patient, and that the "disagreement face" was your way of saying let's talk about this privately. Inform the other therapist that you would simply like them to show you the same consideration.

How do I handle a child who wants to play/cry at every treatment session instead of having their treatment, and refuses to cooperate?

This scenario can play itself out in any practice setting. Depending on how much crying is involved, the level of frustration that you will experience in this scenario can range from very mild annoyance to extremely over-the-top disruption of your patient interaction, and negatively affect the rest of your workday. You must have multiple strategies to address this situation. Otherwise, you will regret it. Uncooperative children have a way of disrupting your day in a way that nothing else can. Here are some suggested strategies to effectively handle this scenario.

- If the child is not the patient, explain to the parent that it may not be a good idea to bring the child next time.

- Make sure the parents bring lots of toys and snacks.

- Just do fun things for the first couple sessions so the child will look forward to their time with you.

- In order to keep the child's attention, be creative in designing activities which are both fun and therapeutic.

- Kids like money, bribe them with pocket change to cooperate during the session. I find that parents really get a kick out of it.

- Keep candy in your pockets, for quick access.

How do I deal with a patient who does not want to see any physical therapist except the one they were working with before, even though I am the only one they can see at the particular time?

It is important to respect and understand the power of the relationship between therapist and patient. You must remember that the patient comes to you in their worst hour of need, exposing their deepest physical vulnerabilities to you while trusting that you will not violate or exploit them in any way. When they have determined that they can truly put their trust in you, and you have determined that you will use your abilities to try and help them, an emotional bond is formed. This bond may or may not be readily apparent, and may or may not be very strong, but it is there. And it is usually strengthened through time. So, when we consider all of these factors, it is not surprising that the patient only wants to be treated by the person he/she has invested themselves into. Our challenge, as physical therapists with a common goal in the improvement of the patient's condition, is to avoid taking it personal and find a way to work through this "touchy" situation while being able to effectively perform our job. Easier said than done? Yes. Can it be done easily? Yes. Here are some ways to do it.

- Listen to their concerns, and then explain to the other therapist did a great job documenting everything about them including their progress and plans for future treatment. Tell them that you will simply be following their plan of care to the letter.

- Ask the patient's usual therapist to tell you anything personal about the patient that you could talk about in order to make them more comfortable with you, and know that you have discussed their condition with their usual therapist in detail, and are very familiar with the plan of treatment.

- Sometimes, patients develop sort of a personal attachment to the therapist who treats them and almost feel as if that therapist "belongs" to them. If you work with the patient's usual therapist on a regular basis, tell the patient that you work with "their therapist" all the time, and you are very familiar with their particular style. You will be doing the same things that "their therapist" was doing in the past.

- Tell the patient that you are a very competent therapist who is treats people with their condition every day. Tell them that you would like them to give you a try just for this one day, and if they still want to see their usual therapist instead, they will have to address it with scheduling.

- If you have seen patients for this therapist in the past or on a regular basis, tell the patient that their usual therapist cannot see them today because of (name the reason), and you that you are the one who usually sees his/her patients when they cannot. Tell them treatment will be exactly the same with only subtle differences in style.

- Sometimes the patient thinks of the new therapist as the "understudy" of the first therapist. Instead of taking it as a personal insult to your knowledge and abilities as a physical therapist, use this to help make the patient more comfortable with being treated by you. If it's just a one-time thing, and you will only be seeing the patient for this one day, tell the patient in a friendly way that you will just be treating them this time, and then they will resume seeing their regular therapist on every session after this. Tell them that you are "almost" as good as their regular therapist, and they are more than welcome to "report how well you did" to the other therapist

130

when they see them next time. Then give them the absolute best treatment you can provide. In the end, you will never be as good as the other therapist in this patient's eyes, but you will be respected, and they will be comfortable enough to allow you to effectively do your job.

How do I deal with a situation where a patient only wants to see me, but I can't see them because of scheduling conflicts or some other reason?

As the great physical therapist that you are, you are bound to find yourself in this scenario throughout your career. Although it can be flattering, it can often become a source of frustration for you, the patient, and the practice facility. It can also lead to the patient unnecessarily avoiding treatment, and thus experiencing worsening of their condition. So how do veteran physical therapists handle this delicate situation? Well, read on.

- Let the patient know in advance that you will not be seeing them that particular day, and personally introduce the therapist who will be seeing them. Tell them that the new therapist is an exceptional PT who you would trust with your own family.

- Tell the other therapist something personal about the patient that only you and the patient knows. Make sure it's something that the patient would not mind you telling other people, such as a funny story he may have told you, etc. Tell the other therapist to relay this story back to the patient so that they will know that you have discussed their condition with the other therapist in detail. This should help the patient feel more comfortable with working with the other therapist.

- Briefly introduce the patient to the therapist who will be treating him at the next session in advance. In this way, your patient won't think that you're just trying to dump them off on another therapist to get rid of them because your tired of them.

- If your office has individual fact sheets about each physical therapist, give one to the patient, telling them you want them to know about the physical therapist is who will be treating them because the therapist will already know who they are by that time.

131

- If your patient is in close proximity to one of the other therapist's patients during therapy session, allow the other patient to brag and rave about the therapist and their skills to your patient. It's good for your patient to hear "at first, I couldn't do this, but now I can't, thanks to my physical therapist, Dr. Johnson". This should help your patient become comfortable with the abilities of the other therapist.

- While interacting with your patient during therapy, include some story of the other therapists interesting accomplishments. For instance, something like "you should have seen the way that patient walked before Dr. Williams, the therapists you will be seeing, started treating him. He is walking so much better now".

How do I deal with a patient who shows racial prejudice and blatant disrespect toward me during treatment, and who makes it known that they would rather be treated by a person of another race, but I am the only PT available?

There are thousands upon thousands of physical therapists in the world today, and they come from all over the world and consist of many races and backgrounds. Unfortunately, there are a handful of people in this world who consider that a bad thing, and would like to impose their views upon you if you are of a different race that they are. It places you in an awkward situation which you were probably not trained in school to handle. Have no fear, suggestions are here:

- First, be absolutely sure that the person is really a racist-type person, and is really attempting to tell you that they want to be treated by a therapist of another race, because there is nothing worse than accusing someone of racism and being wrong.

- Be very professional while explaining the obvious to them, that quality of care is no different between physical therapists of different races. But if they stand firm refer them to another therapist.

- If you are indeed sure of the patient's racism, stop, think, and figure out what the most distinguished person would do in this situation, and then do it.

- Quietly confront the issue with the patient in a private place. Tell them that your goal is to provide the absolute best PT service that one can have, but your sensing hostility toward you for no apparent reason, and ask them for the reason. If the patient denies, take them for their word, apologize, and move on.

- I would give the patient the option of staying and giving me the opportunity of providing treatment, but if they decided not to, I show them the door.

- Let your supervisor know about it, and ask for that patient to be quietly removed from your daily patient schedule so that you just won't have to interact with the person.

- Be frank and completely honest. Tell the patient that you are feeling negativity toward you. Do not waste your time attempting to ask the patient if the problem is because they harbor negative racial feelings toward you, because chances are that they will probably be untruthful anyway. Simply inform the patient that you will be making sure they are treated by another therapist. Then go straight to your supervisor and inform them of the situation. Note: You can also go to your supervisor first, but then it would not show your level of independent problem solving.

- As soon as you have decided that the patient does indeed desire to be treated by a person of another race, excuse yourself in a very professional way and immediately inform your supervisor. A good supervisor will address the problem at once. Allow the supervisor to determine the next course of action.

- If there are other therapists on staff, choose which therapist the patient would most likely be most comfortable with. Then explain the situation to the therapist, and ask if they would like to trade patients with you for the remainder of that patients scheduled sessions.

- Explain to the patient that you as a therapist, and the facility for which you work (hospital, outpatient, etc.) do not discriminate in treatment of any patient based on race. Tell them that it would also be illegal to do so. After informing the patient of your stance, allow them to decide what they would like to do from that point. Note: You **MUST** be absolutely sure that the patient's desire to be treated by another person is strictly due to racial preference. You cannot risk falsely accusing a patient based on your own personal feeling. You must actually hear the words come from the patient's mouth.

How do I deal with a patient whose injuries were apparently due to physical abuse by a spouse or parent, but who tries to conceal the truth?

Whoa! Did we really include this scenario? You bet we did, and it is because it happens. This is an extremely delicate situation, and can be scary for the patient and intimidating for the physical therapist. Furthermore, if not addressed appropriately, can lead to a horrible outcome for all parties involved. It has happened to some of your PT colleagues, so consider their advice below on how to approach this scenario.

- Get general facts, report them to any on-staff social worker if available, and let them take it from there.

- This is a case to take to your supervisors. Just make sure you point to specific and objective reasons that you suspect physical abuse.

- If there are no mental or social health workers available, try to make the patient comfortable enough to discuss the truth, and then give them options on seeking help.

- Be completely straightforward and honest. Ask "are these bruises from fighting?", "has someone been physically hurting you?", or "please don't be offended, but I noticed the bruises, and have seen patients in physically abusive situations. I am not saying that you are, but if you need help, I have resources".

- Don't mention physical abuse. Instead, talk about how they sustained the bruises. Document exactly what the patient says. Then during a normal conversation on the next visit, have the patient repeat the same story, and compare to the previous story. Inform the patient of any inconsistencies in the story, and tell them that inconsistencies are a red flag, and doesn't mean that they are being physically abused, but that it does require that you to take further action for their safety. Then refer them to the appropriate health care professional.

How do I deal with a patient who comes for treatment while apparently intoxicated with alcohol or drugs?

Not only is this scenario fairly common, especially in an outpatient setting, but it can be very dangerous to everyone involved, and render your treatment interventions ineffective at best. The thing about this scenario is that when addressing it, things can go south…fast…real fast. When you find yourself in this situation, make your life easier by considering the advice of other physical therapists who have been there, themselves.

- First, investigate the reasons behind their actions. Make sure they are actually intoxicated before accusing them of such a thing. If the patient is slurring speech and their walking is unstable and uncoordinated, it could easily be due to a neurologic condition such as CVA. It would be very embarrassing and unprofessional to accuse a patient who is having or has had a CVA of being drunk. They could also have a combination of problems such as a pre-existing balance dysfunction, and showing effects from high dose prescription pain medication. Don't jump the gun on your suspicions because if you are wrong, it could be catastrophic for you, and will only further a negative perception that your age and lack of experience makes you less of a physical therapist.

- You must be perfectly honest. Make sure the patient is in a private area where your conversation won't be heard by others. Begin with letting the patient know that your job involves guarding the safety of your patients. Tell them that you would not be doing your job, and wouldn't be the great therapist that you are if you did not act on your observations.

Then, ask the patient how they feel, and tell them what you are noticing. Tell them what it looks like. Finally, tell the patient that your concerned for their safety and also the safety of other patients. If the patient confesses to being intoxicated, DO NOT make them feel bad about it. They may not have thought about the consequences, and had no ill will about what they are doing.

- Let the patient know that you are obligated to provide them treatment and in a professional manner and they are obligated to present themselves in a manner in which is acceptable for treatment. Advise them that you are unable to treat them today and reschedule them for another visit and make sure to let them know that if they show up in the same disposition that you will not be able to treat them then either. Explain to them that this is not just for their safety, but for the peace and safety of everyone in the facility.

- Simply inform the patient that you will need 100% of their attention, and have to cancel the days treatment and for reasons of safety.

- If the patient demonstrates an obvious decrease in coordination and balance, inform them that you noticed that they had poor coordination and difficulty maintaining their balance, and tell them that you can tell that they had a "couple drinks" because you smell alcohol on them. Tell them that you are just concerned that the balance problem may be due to a worsening of their condition, but that it may be due to alcohol instead. Then inform the patient that you will be cancelling today's session so that you can compare their balance today with their balance at next session to determine if its due to the alcohol or due to a worsening in their condition. Tell them that it is important that they not have any alcohol in their system when they return. At the next session, if their balance appears normal, and they do not appear intoxicated, tell them that it means the balance problem was due to alcohol, and they can no longer have any alcohol in their system during a physical therapy session, because it interferes with your ability to assess their balance and coordination.

Tips on treating a mentally ill patient who has a physical injury?

People who sustain physical illness almost always have other pre-existing conditions that complicate delivery of treatment interventions, and one of these conditions can be mental illness. It may not be something you will see every day, so handling this scenario can be somewhat difficult. Nevertheless, it is important to handle it well. Here are some suggestions on how to do just that.

- Try to make sure there is a family member or personal caretaker present to help deal with any unusual behavior that they may demonstrate.

"Reorganize your schedule to allow more time to be spent with this patient". Eric Wanner. PT, DPT, OCS. West Palm Beach, FL

- Family members love to play an interactive role in helping their loved one. So, tell the family member that you are "recruiting" them as a team partner in the patient's treatment, and you will need them to help you navigate around the patient's unique mental limitations that you are unaware of. You and the patient's family member will make a great team, and all will go well.

- Be very patient, speak up, speak very clearly, and in a very friendly tone.

- Modify their treatment based on their personal cognitive disability. For example, if they have difficulty following orders, give one order at a time, and make the task very simple and uncomplicated. Or if the patient has an attention deficit, divide your communication into short intervals, and touch the patient frequently to keep their attention.

How do I deal with a situation where a patient's health insurance runs out before they should be discharged?

This scenario plays itself out every single day in every physical therapy practice facility throughout the entire United States, and is a daily challenge, in one way or another to all physical therapists. Welcome to the United States healthcare system, where insurance companies dictate your patient's healthcare. This should not be a challenge in this country, but it is, so instead of complaining about it, here are methods to deal with it.

- Be honest, and inform them that their insurance won't allow you to treat them anymore, then issue two or three progressively increasing stages of home exercises which they can progressively advance from one stage to the next as they feel ready.

- Discuss the situation with the patient, inform them of the out-of-pocket option, and then suggest spreading out PT sessions to accommodate their finances.

- When you discharge them, make sure they understand that they can call you anytime at the clinic if they have any questions or concerns about their condition or home exercises.

- If they will benefit from continued exercise, be sure to have a list of local workout gyms which they can join. Make sure there are names of contact persons on the list who know you or your clinic.

- Talk with your supervisor about developing a program which will allow the patient and future patients to continue exercising at the clinic pro bono or for a small fee.

How do I deal with a situation where I am romantically interested in a patient, and we both seem to want to further pursue the idea?

This is a very serious matter because it tests your maturity and conviction to the honor of your profession. Further, moving forward in a situation such as this could be against ethical guidelines. Ultimately, the decision is up to you, but you never want to be an embarrassment to the profession. So here are some suggestions by other therapists.

- Step one: Do not pursue. Step two: Refer to step one.

- Wait until after the patient is discharged before taking even the smallest steps in this direction.

- If you and the patient cannot wait, transfer the patient to another therapist, let your supervisor know, and never treat that person in professional capacity from that point onward.

- Politely, but firmly inform the patient that whether you want to or not, the issue is completely out of the question because you DO NOT get involved with your patients. And then stick to what you have said.

- Explain the situation to your supervisor, and ask if there are any company policies regarding this situation. Also ask them for their opinion on the situation. If they are not against to the idea, and it is not against company policy, go for it. But only fraternize with your new romantic interest after work, and remain professional at all times during work hours.

How do I deal with the patient who only wants physical therapy in order to get a massage?

Ahhh yes, the old "massage issue". Believe it or not, this kind of situation does occur a lot, especially if you are particularly good with your manual skills. Here is a classic scenario: the patient has a diagnosis of lumbar muscle strain. Your treatment interventions include moist heat to loosen and relax soft tissue, electrical stimulation for pain control, therapeutic exercise to improve muscle strength and posture and improve soft tissue extensibility, and manual soft tissue mobilization/ massage to improve soft tissue mobility and decrease painful muscle spasm. You notice the patient always makes excuses to avoid exercise and all other interventions except the massage because "everything else makes the pain worse". You make exceptions on a few instances, and the next thing you know, massage is the only treatment you are providing for that patient. Further, the patient is either progressing slow or not at all because they are not receiving proper treatment for their condition. Does this sound familiar? If so, here are some suggestions by others who have found themselves in similar situations.

- Explain to them that even though massage feels good, it is not helping to resolve their condition. Then give them a copy of a list of local massage therapists that you have on hand for this type of situation.

- Perform a re-evaluation, and obtain objective measurements of strength, pain, posture, ROM, etc. If they are not making adequate progress, tell them so. Then inform the patient that you will need to discharge them from physical therapy if improvements are not seen within the next couple of sessions. Once they realize that this means no more massage for them, they may decide to bite the bullet and tolerate the other treatment interventions, and start improving.

- Educate the patient about how each of the other less desirable treatment interventions help improve their condition. Help them understand that they will improve faster when you can address the problem from all angles.

- Remind the patient that you are a physical therapist, and proceed to tell them what it is that you do. Then tell them that massage is provided by a massage therapist, and they will need to schedule an appointment with one in order to receive massage therapy.

- Explain the difference between a massage therapist and physical therapist. Be specific on education, scope of practice, and difference between therapeutic massage and "comfort" massage.

- Choose one of the following phrases to tell the patient: "this type of massage is not necessarily meant to make you feel better, but to loosen soft tissue enough so that the other aspects of physical therapy can be helpful" "massage alone will not improve your condition, it just happens to feel good while its being performed"

- Have business cards of local therapy facilities on hand, and give one to the patient saying, " I can refer you to a massage therapist who will be happy to spend lots of time with you performing massage if you would like, but we are here for physical therapy"

- Explain to the patient the specific reason behind performing therapeutic massage or soft tissue mobilization.

- Tell the patient that your job is to facilitate the fastest and most efficient recovery possible, and performing massage as the only intervention would not make that happen, and would mean that you were not performing your job well. Tell them that you are very serious about making them better, and ask them to allow you to do your job and show them how good you are.

- If all else fails, explain to the patient that most insurance companies will reject payment if massage is the only treatment being performed. Then they will be responsible for full payment, which could be very costly to them.

How do I deal with the patient who has fully recovered from the injury for which they were referred to me, and only wants physical therapy in order to use me as a "free personal trainer" for fitness/body sculpting, etc.?

This type of situation usually occurs in an outpatient orthopedic setting. It is, in fact, a source of frustration for the physical therapist, and disrupts the continuity and flow of that therapist's treatment plan. You, as the therapist may feel as if the patient is attempting to manipulate you, but don't want to cause friction with the patient, especially after such a great rehab outcome. The good news is that it probably means you did an excellent job with this patient. The bad news is that your job is not over. You have to transition the person from recovering patient to rehabilitated patient. Here are a few suggestions.

- Have business cards of local therapy facilities on hand, and give one to the patient saying "I can refer you to a personal trainer who will be happy to work with you on a personal training level".

- If the patient does not have a physical condition, and objective measurements do not show deficits, inform the patient that they are not a candidate for physical therapy, refer them to an exercise gym, and discharge them from physical therapy.

- Inform the patient that their health insurance will not cover general exercise.

- Inform them that since insurance won't pay for simply working out, they may be responsible for paying thousands of dollars out of the pocket.

"Suggest that a workout gym may be more cost effective for them, and then refer them to a local exercise gym". Danladi Whitten, MPT. Washington, DC

- Some outpatient PT facilities are starting to institute exercise programs for patients who have progressed through PT and have been discharged. These patients then pay a small fee to use the PT gym as a workout facility. If your facility has this program, utilize it, if not make a strong request to your supervisors. Tell them it's a great way to ease the discharge process for the patient, and it generates more income (they should be receptive when you mention generating more income).

- If you are not a certified athletic or personal trainer, get certified. Then, these patients will be automatic candidates for increased revenue for you on a part-time basis during your off-work hours either at your facility or contract with another fitness gym. When these patients suggest that they would like to workout give them the option of paying you for your time and expertise.

How do I deal with a supervisor who is overloading me with too many patients:

In researching for this text, this situation seemed to come up as often as any subject. It also seems to stir a lot of passion. This is because good therapists are passionate about their job. They don't like rushing when applying their clinical reasoning skills and when performing their duties. Most therapists felt that adequate time is necessary and must be taken in order to perform physical therapy. Otherwise, mistakes occur, ideas are missed, and actions performed poorly. This in turn, takes away from your abilities to perform your duties, and makes you worse off as a physical therapist for it. Here are some suggestions in case you find yourself in this all too well-known scenario.

- First, make a consorted effort to manage the problem independently. If you then decide that there are still too many patients, be candid with your supervisor and inform them that the patient load is too much for you to handle at this time (if you are a new PT, they should be more than willing to listen and help where they can).

- Call the your local state chapter of the APTA or the state governing bodies to determine if there are any local laws that govern the number of patients you are allowed to see per hour. Some states that a restriction on the number of patients a physical therapist is allowed to treat within a given time frame.

- Apply for other physical therapy positions where this problem does not exist. Once you have solid prospects, kindly and respectfully explain the situation to your supervisor and give them your two-week notice. If they are amendable to making change, they will immediately do so, and you can turn the prospect down. If not, they will accept your resignation, freeing you to accept the better position. Problem solved.

- Suggest several alternative solutions to your supervisor such as spreading the patient load among other therapists until you

143

become more comfortable with a heavy load, assigning more help in the form of aids or PT techs to perform non-skilled part of treatment such as ultrasound and moist heat modalities, or working a longer day while spreading the patient appointments out so that you may have enough time with each patient before the next one comes.

- Research other local PT facilities similar to the one you work at and compare the number of patients per therapist. If the number is significantly lower on average, keep the information as proof and show it to your supervisor.

- Research local laws and city ordinances which may limit the number of patients a physical therapist may see with any given time frame. If your supervisor is not compliant with the law, he/she may not know. So simply inform him/her. You should then see results immediately.

Must-have physical therapy reference texts:

As a new physical therapist, it is imperative for you to start building your library of clinical reference texts. The more extensive the library, the better for you. Start by purchasing one at a time until you have amassed a large library for professional reference. Here are some texts suggested by other veteran therapists:

- Grants Anatomy
- Flash Anatomy by Bryan Edwards
- Clinical Musculoskeletal Anatomy by Neal Pratt
- The Rehabilitation Specialists Handbook by Jules Rothstein
- Pocket Guide to Musculoskeletal Assessment by Richard Baxter
- Pharmacology for Health professionals by Sally roach
- Primary care for the Physical Therapist by William Boissonault
- Fundamentals of Musculoskeletal Imaging by Lynn Mckinnis
- Contraindication in Physical Rehabilitation by Mitchell Batavia
- Mosby's PDQ for Massage by Sandy fritz
- Neuromusculoskeletal Examination and Assessment by Nicola Petty

- Maitland's Peripheral Manipulation by Elly Hengeveld and Kevin Banks
- Maitland's Vertebral Manipulation by Elly Hengeveld, Kevin banks, and Kay English
- Manipulation of the Spine Thorax and Pelvis by Peter Gibbons
- Clinical Examination of the Shoulder by Todd S. Ellenbecker
- Clinical Orthopedic Rehabilitation by S. Brent Brotzman
- Clinical Anatomy of the Lumbar Spine and sacrum by Nikolai Bogduk
- Greve's Modern Manual Therapy by Jeffrey D. Boyling and Gwendolen A. Jull
- Differential Examination and Treatment of Movement Disorders in Manual Therapy by Robert Pfund
- Stroke Rehabilitation by janet Carr, and Robert Shephard
- Diagnosis and Treatment of Movement Impairment syndromes by Shirley A. Sahrmann
- Physical Therapy of the Shoulder by Robert Donatelli
- Pocket guide to Musculoskeletal Assessment by Richard E. Baxter
- Physical Rehabilitation of the Injured Athlete by J. Andrews, G. Harrelson, and K. Wilk
- Cranial Manipulation Theory and practice by Leon Chaitow
- Orthopedic Clinical Examination: an Evidence based Approach for PTs by Joshua Cleland
- Orthotics and Prosthetics in rehabilitation by Michelle M. Lusardi and Caroline C. Nielson
- Pharmacology for Physical therapists by Barbara Gladson
- Physiotherapy Practice in residential Aged Care by Jennifer C. Nitz and Susan R. Hourigan
- Sports Injuries Diagnosis and Management by Christopher Norris
- Rehabilitation for the Postsurgical Orthopedic Patient by Lisa Maxey and Jim Magnusson
- Joint Mobilization Manipulation by Susan Edmond
- Direct Release Myofascial Technique by Michael Stanborough
- Functional Outcomes documentation for Rehabilitation by Lori Quinn and James Gordon

Suggestion for functional goals.

Functional goals are one of the most important parts of the initial evaluation and re-evaluation process, and are necessary in order to implement treatment intervention strategies. Further, third party insurance companies routinely deny payment if goals are not stated clearly. These goals should be functional, have a definite timeframe for completion, and be measurable. Here are a few suggestions from other veteran therapists that may help you when designing a plan of care after evaluating a patient. I must stress that this is not a cheat sheet to simply be copied word for word, but suggestions for you to modify as needed based on your patient's particular situation. Also, while modifying the following suggested goals, remember that each goal should have a time frame for completion and be measurable. It should also be relevant to the condition at hand and be attainable. One way to remember all of the components of a goal is to remember the acronym "SMART". It stands for goals that are Specific, Measurable, Attainable, Relevant, and Time-based. So, think "smart" while using these following suggested goals to help create your own.

- **Cervical:**
  ✓ Pt will have enough ROM to be able to rotate head without difficulty in order to drive
  ✓ Pt will be able to sleep at night without being awakened by pain
  ✓ Pt's cervical posture will improve enough to allow him to sit and watch entire movie without difficulty
  ✓ Pt will have no longer have difficulty flexing the neck and looking down when buttoning her shirt
  ✓ Pt will no longer require the use of cervical collar/neck brace
  ✓ Pt will be able to extend cervical spine enough to shave under chin
  ✓ Pt will be able to properly and effectively stretch his own neck independently to relieve pain/stiffness
  ✓ Pt will be able to use proper cervical posture when using computer workstation at work
  ✓ Pt will be able to don/doff buttonless shirt without difficulty
  ✓ Pt will be able to nod head yes/no without painful difficulty
  ✓ Pt will have full ROM in all planes of motion at the cervical spine in order to be able to return to birdwatching hobby as he did prior to injury.
  ✓ Radicular sx and paresthesia radiating from the neck will decrease enough for patient to hold a plate of food without dropping it on the floor.

- ✓ Patient will perform ADLs involving overhead activities such as reaching into overhead cabinets without difficulty or assistance.
- ✓ Pt will be able to decrease the number of pillows required for him to comfortably sleep to the number he used prior to the injury.
- ✓ Pt will have a significant decrease in pain which will allow him to discontinue sleeping in lounge chair and start sleeping in normal bed
- ✓ Pt will be able to return to work and perform work activities without difficulty.
- ✓ Pt will be able to bend forward at the trunk when picking up items from the floor without limitation due to neck pain.
- ✓ Pt will be able to maneuver her neck functionally in order to drink water from water fountain at work with no difficulty.
- ✓ Pt will be able to hold her neck in a single position for more than one hour without difficulty as is required when reading her school textbooks for exams.
- ✓ Pt will be able to hold head still enough to brush teeth without difficulty.

- **Shoulder:**
- ✓ Patient will have enough ROM to be able to reach into overhead kitchen cabinets without difficulty
- ✓ Patient will have enough strength to be able to throw a baseball without significant difficulty
- ✓ Pt will have enough ROM to be able to don shirt or jacket without significant difficulty
- ✓ Pt will full ROM in order to allow him to perform his regular work activities involving use of the shoulder
- ✓ Pt will have normal shoulder strength in order for him to be able to lift his 2 year old son
- ✓ Pt will have a significant decrease in pain which will allow him to sleep through the night without being awakened by pain
- ✓ Pt will able to use shoulder properly when removing a gallon of milk from the refrigerator
- ✓ Pt will be able to demonstrate independence with stretching exercises in order to address future recurrence of tightness/pain in the shoulder.
- ✓ Pt will demonstrate normal shoulder posture in order to perform ADLs and work activities without aggravating the injury or causing re-injury.

- ✓ Pt will be able to reach behind her in order to fasten/unfasten bra
- ✓ Pt will be able to reach behind his back without difficulty in order to reach wallet in rear pocket.
- ✓ Pt will have enough shoulder ROM to allow him to wash hair without difficulty or assistance.
- ✓ Pt will be able to return to his hobby of playing basketball without difficulty.
- ✓ Pt will be able to discontinue use of shoulder sling without an increase in pain.
- ✓ Pt will be able to use shoulder properly when carrying groceries
- ✓ Pt will have enough ROM and strength to pass competency skills test as required by his employer in order for him to return to work.
- ✓ Pt will be able to use shoulder properly when transitioning from supine to sitting position
- ✓ Pt will have 5/5 shoulder strength and Full ROM in all planes of motion as is necessary for functional use of shoulder during household cleaning activities without difficulty.
- ✓ Pt will be able to tolerate manual therapy in order to improve ROM to a functional level.
- ✓ Pt will have full ROM and strength, and pain will decrease enough for him to return to rock climbing hobby as he was before the injury.

- **Elbow:**
- ✓ Patient's decrease in pain will be enough to allow him to throw a baseball to his son
- ✓ Patient will have enough strength to be able to close car door without difficulty
- ✓ Patient will have enough elbow strength to don clothes without difficulty
- ✓ Patient will be able to fully flex elbow without difficulty in order to shave
- ✓ Patient will have enough elbow strength to carry his suitcase for work
- ✓ Patient will have enough elbow strength to lift objects as required for work
- ✓ Patient will be able to properly use elbow when transitioning from sitting to standing position
- ✓ Patient will have enough ROM to use elbow properly while cooking

- ✓ Patient will have enough ROM to be able to perform benchpress exercise during his usual workout
- ✓ Patient will be able to use elbow properly when steering his vehicle while driving
- ✓ Patient will be able to use elbow properly when perform work activities
- ✓ Patient will be able to bend elbow enough to comb hair
- ✓ Patient will be able to properly use elbow when picking up objects from the floor
- ✓ Patient will be able to properly use elbow to reach overhead shelves
- ✓ Patient will demonstrate ability to carry bags of groceries without difficulty
- ✓ Patient will be able to use elbow properly when controlling gear shift while driving
- ✓ Patient will be able to use elbow functionally when lifting his/her child
- ✓ Patient will be able to use elbow properly when reaching into rear pants pocket
- ✓ Patient will be able to properly use elbow when opening and closing doors
- ✓ Pt will be able to remove a gallon of milk from refrigerator
- ✓ Patient will a have decrease in pain which will allow proper use of elbow when painting his home
- ✓ Patient will demonstrate independence w/elbow stretch exercises for temporary relief of pain/tightness

- • **Wrist:**
- ✓ Patient will have enough strength to hold a one gallon container of milk without difficulty
- ✓ Patient will have enough supination ROM to be able to turn a doorknob in order to open door.
- ✓ Patient will have enough wrist and hand dexterity to use a pen to write without difficulty.
- ✓ Patient will be able to button shirt when dressing
- ✓ Patient will be able to use wrist properly when shaving
- ✓ Patient will be able to use wrist properly when combing hair
- ✓ Patient will be able to use wrist/hand properly when opening car door
- ✓ Patient will be able to use wrist properly when stirring a pot of food while cooking
- ✓ Patient will be able to hold a pot/skillet of food without difficulty

- ✓ Patient will be able to perform all work activities involving use of wrist without difficulty
- ✓ Patient will be able to play tennis as he did prior to injury
- ✓ Patient will be able to use wrist properly when ironing clothes
- ✓ Patient will be able to use wrist properly when performing household chores such as cleaning sink
- ✓ Patient will be able to use wrist properly when opening a drawer
- ✓ Patient will be able to use wrist functionally when working on his car
- ✓ Patient will have functional use of wrist when typing on computer keyboard
- ✓ Patient will be able to use wrist without difficulty when mowing the lawn
- ✓ Patient will have enough ROM at the wrist to perform pushups as he did prior to injury/surgery
- ✓ Patient will have enough wrist strength to twist off a tight jar lid as he did before injury
- ✓ Patient will have enough wrist dexterity to use wrist properly when bathing

- • **Back:**
- ✓ Pt will have enough mobility of the lumbar spine in order to bend at the trunk while standing to tie shoes
- ✓ Pt will have able to tolerate standing for eight continuous hours without pain in order to perform work duties as his job requires.
- ✓ Pt will have enough ROM in the lumbar spine to transition from sitting to standing position without pain
- ✓ Decrease in LBP/stiffness will be enough to allow pt to sit for two hours in order to drive out of town
- ✓ Pt will be able to demonstrate independence with proper stooping posture in order to decreased exacerbation of LBP
- ✓ Pt will be able to transition from supine to sit without assistance in order to have independent bed mobility
- ✓ Pain and stiffness will decrease enough to allow pt to return to previous level of recreational activity such as playing basketball
- ✓ Pt will be able to swim as he did before the back injury
- ✓ Pt will have enough trunk strength to be able to lift her 12 month old child without difficulty ROM in lumbar spine will improve to normal in order for pt to be able to lean forward to work on his vehicle

✓ Pt will have 5/5 lumbar strength in order to be able to wear backpack filled with books as he normally does
✓ LBP/stiffness will decrease to 0-2/10 in order for pt to ride bicycle without difficulty
✓ Pt will demonstrate normal trunk posture without flexion at the trunk in order to ambulate without difficulty
✓ Pt will experience an improvement to normal trunk strength and posture in order to eliminate the need for the use of an assistive device ambulate independently.
✓ Pt will be able to sleep for entire night without waking due to back pain
✓ Pt will be able to demonstrate independence with home exercise program in order to temporarily decrease exacerbations of LBP and stiffness
✓ Pt will be able to independently transition to and from car in order to be able to drive.
✓ Lumbar strength and ROM will improve to normal limits in order for pt to return to prior level of workout regimen without difficulty.
✓ Lumbar strength will improve to normal in order for patient to be able to dispose of bags of trash
✓ Lumbar ROM will improve enough to allow patient to use vacuum cleaner while cleaning the home.

- **Hip:**
✓ Pt will have enough mobility to transition from sitting to standing position without difficulty
✓ Pt will have enough strength in the hip to ride a bike for ten minutes without difficulty
✓ Pt will have a pain decrease enough to allow him/her to walk up and down a flight of stairs at least once a day without significant difficulty
✓ Pt will show an improvement in balance enough to allow him/her to ambulate for 60 feet without an assistive device and without significant difficulty.
✓ Pt will be able to sit for more than one hour without stiffness and difficulty
✓ Pt will be able to return to playing softball without difficulty while running the bases
✓ Pt will be able to independently move involved leg when transitioning from supine position to sitting on side of bed

- ✓ Pt will be able to demonstrate independence with stretch exercises in order to relieve temporary tightness and pain in the hip.
- ✓ Pt will experience a decrease in pain and increase in strength and ROM to normal limits in order to be able to don and doff pants without difficulty
- ✓ Pt will be able to use involved leg to operate the clutch mechanism of his manual transmission car without difficulty in order to drive.
- ✓ Pt will be able to squat without difficulty in the manner which is required for work performance.
- ✓ Pt will be able to stoop at the hip without difficulty when picking up items from the ground.
- ✓ Pt will be able to squat low enough to tie shoes without difficulty
- ✓ Pt will no longer experience more than 2/10 morning pain/stiffness after waking, and will be able to stand and walk immediately after waking from sleep in the morning.
- ✓ Pt will be able to transition to and from seated position in her car without difficulty.
- ✓ Pt will be able to use the step board feature of her trunk in order to climb into her vehicle without difficulty.
- ✓ Pt will be able to safely climb into tub without assistance or difficulty
- ✓ Pt's weightbearing tolerance will improve to the point where he will be able to stand for more than one hour without difficulty
- ✓ Pt will be able to return to using the elliptical machine at his workout gym without difficulty
- ✓ Pt will be able to sit in a modest comfortable position with involved leg crossed over the other as she did before the injury.

- **Knee:**
- ✓ Pt will be able to demonstrate full knowledge of prescribed knee strengthening HEP in order to perform home exercises without assistance.
- ✓ Pt will be able to ascend and descend a flight of ten stairs without assistance or difficulty
- ✓ Pt will be able to squat in order to perform work activities involving this position.

- ✓ Pt will be able to sit for 30 minutes with 90 degree knee flexion without experiencing significant pain and difficulty walking upon standing.
- ✓ Pt will be able to return to usual every day running regimen of 1 mile without difficulty
- ✓ Pt will be able to stand for more than one hour without sitting.
- ✓ Pt will be able to discontinue use of cane as assistive device, and without demonstrating antalgic and dysfunctional gait pattern.
- ✓ Pt will be able to tolerate full weightbearing through both knees without difficulty immediately after waking in the morning.
- ✓ Pt will be able to demonstrate proper and safe use of crutch/cane/walker
- ✓ Pt will be able to transition from sitting to standing position with full weightbearing tolerance without difficulty
- ✓ Pt will swim 5 full laps in pool as she was able to do regularly before the injury and subsequent surgery.
- ✓ Pt will Pt will be able to sleep throughout a full night without being awakened by pain
- ✓ Pt will be able to demonstrate independence with stretch exercise program in order to address recurrence of dysfunctional pain/tightness in the knee.
- ✓ Pt will have full ROM throughout the knee in order to sit in cross-legged position as she did before the initial injury.
- ✓ Pt will have normal knee strength in order to be able to bend at the knees without difficulty when lifting a heavy item.
- ✓ Pt will be able to ride his bicycle for 3 miles as he did before surgery.
- ✓ Pt will be able to climb into tub safely and without difficulty.
- ✓ Pt will be able to use legs properly to push or pull 100 pound cases along the floor as is required for his occupation.
- ✓ Pt will be able to climb into her truck without difficulty in order to drive
- ✓ Pt will have no difficulty when using involved leg to apply the clutch while driving.

- **Foot:**
- ✓ Pt will be able to bear full weight on involved foot without difficulty
- ✓ Pt will be able to ambulate without assistive device
- ✓ Pt will be able to ascend a flight of ten stairs with only the use of handrail as support

- ✓ Pt will be able to descend a flight of ten stairs without difficulty or assistive device
- ✓ Pt will be able to apply the brake and accelerator pedals without difficulty while driving
- ✓ Pt will be able to wear his usual shoes without difficulty
- ✓ Pt will be able to stand for 8 hours as is a requirement for his employment.
- ✓ Pt will be able to return to hobby of running 1 mile every other day without difficulty, as he did prior to injury.
- ✓ Pt will be able to wear shoes with half-inch heel without complaints of difficulty with ambulation due to discomfort.
- ✓ Pt will be able to discontinue use of ankle immobilizer with her doctor's approval
- ✓ Pt will be able to discontinue use of assistive device with his doctor's approval;
- ✓ Pt will be able to ambulate safely and without antalgic gait
- ✓ Pt will be able to stand on toes as is a necessary requirement for his job
- ✓ Pt will be able to safely ambulate without shoes
- ✓ Pt will be able to demonstrate proper icing technique in order to independently decrease recurrence of swelling/edema.
- ✓ Pt will be able to demonstrate full independence with home exercise program, including stretches in order to decrease dysfunctional pain and stiffness.
- ✓ Pt will be able to ride his bicycle without difficulty resulting from ankle pain, weakness, swelling, or pain.
- ✓ Pt will be able to grocery shop for one hour without leaning on shopping cart for support.
- ✓ Pt will be able to sleep for the entire night without being awakened by pain
- ✓ Pt will be able to squat while standing on toes as in necessary when loading the dryer while doing laundry at home.

What do I do when a patient acquires questionable information about treatment for their particular condition (from internet, books, infomercials, etc.), and now believes he/she is qualified to instruct me on how to perform my job?

Part of your job as a therapist is to educate the patient about his/her condition in order to equip them with the tools that will allow them to be an active participant in their own recovery and rehabilitation. The more information that the patient has, the less you have to teach. However, it is important to know that in this day and age of information technology, access to information is available to everyone, and the validity of the information and the reliability of the sources can be very questionable, especially to the layperson who does not have your knowledge base.

"Honestly listen to their ideas, evaluate them for appropriateness, and let them know which theories/idea you agree with and which ideas you don't and why". Brett Rice, MPT, FAAOMPT. New Market MD

- Google their injury/condition on your smart phone, and pick out the clearly incorrect and false information that shows up in the search results. Also show them some of the correct information, and explain to them how difficult it is to determine which is good information and which is bad information, and how disastrous it would be for them if they chose the wrong information.

- Don't go with the "I have this degree and you don't speech". It only makes you look as if you are trying to prove something that you can't.

- Ask a veteran physical therapist to tell you a good story of the disastrous outcome of when a patient attempted to self-treat themselves based on internet information. Tell the same story

155

to the patient, and explain to them that you are here to make sure that horrible outcome doesn't happen to them.

- Tell the patient that its good to look up information on the internet regarding treatment of their injury/condition, and that it shows that they are an active participant in their own treatment. Tell them that your inspired by their efforts, but to just run it by you before they implement it.

- Congratulate the patient for being pro-active with their own health, but inform them that they must retrieve their information from legitimate sources, and then give them some suggestions such as web MD or suggest medical magazines such as Men's Health.

How do I deal with a patient who seems to have a legitimate problem and is a candidate for PT, but exaggerates the sx for any reason?

Your patient presents to you for an initial evaluation, and is barely able to ambulate even with a 4-wheel walker. All objective tests and measures confirm the diagnosis of difficulty with ambulation. After the evaluation is completed, although still demonstrating an obvious dysfunctional gait pattern, the patient's ambulation strikingly improves on their way out of the exam room. Once the patient notices that you are watching them, they immediately begin to ambulate as they did initially. Clearly, this patient appears to be exaggerating their condition, but they also clearly have the condition in question. Considering the fact that the degree of exaggeration varies from subtle to over the top, it is fair to say that this is a fairly common occurrence This can be a very frustrating scenario that unnecessarily wastes your valuable time as a physical therapist. However, as so many scenarios in this text, this is a very touchy situation because though the sheer dishonesty makes you want to punch a hole in the wall, and the idea of wasting your time is not something is particularly attractive to you, there are ethical considerations involved, and you are expected to treat this patient for the very real condition that they have. Ugh! Let's find out how veteran physical Therapists handle this kind of scenario.

- Concentrate on treating the patient based on objective findings more than treating them for their subjective complaints.

- Take note of the possible reasons the patient may be exaggerating (personal injury lawsuit, sympathy, time off from work, etc.). Be honest with them, and tell them that although you are certain of some of their injuries, the degree of some of their reported symptoms do not exactly match their actual physical signs. Inform the patient that exaggerating will not help them achieve their objective, and will only make things worse because it decreases their credibility and makes it more difficult to treat the very real symptoms that they do have.

- Show empathy, but do not feed into the exaggerated complaints because this will probably cause the patient to continue the same or even increase the level of exaggeration, and will foster an unproductive relationship between you and the patient.

- If the reason for exaggerating symptoms appear to be for financial gain, such as a person involved in a motor vehicle accident who is currently in legal litigation to be compensated for their injuries, be aware that there is a relatively increased chance that some degree of exaggeration may be at play. Make your interventions based ONLY on objective measurements.

How do I deal with a patient who does not have any symptoms or signs of a condition for which PT is necessary, and who appears to be faking/lying about his problems for any reason?

This scenario is similar to the previous one, but the answer is much simpler, discharge the patient immediately. The problem here is how do you do this in the most appropriate manner without things getting awkward and weird? Once again, let's go to the veteran PTs for the answer.

- Don't assume that the patient is not being truthful without thoroughly investigating your suspicions. If you are absolutely certain that the patient is not being honest about their reported symptoms, explain the situation to your lead physical therapist or direct supervisor. They will advise from that point.

- Use objective date to back up clinical decisions.

- That is why there are objective measurements. After a thorough initial evaluation, inform the patient that you cannot identify any problems using objective measurements, so you can't treat what you can't see. Make recommendations to follow-up with a health professional that may be appropriate for them, including their referring physician if there is one.

- Document your FINDINGS, not your personal suspicions

- Inform the patient that treatment will be based on your FINDINGS

- Contact and inform the referring physician if your findings suggest that there is no problem

How do I deal with the "clingy" patient without hurting their feelings?

Since physical therapists spend more time with patients than most other health professionals, patients tend to become emotionally attached to us. This in turn allows us to interact with the patient on a deeper and more involved level than other healthcare professionals. However, some patients are more emotionally "needy" than others, and expect you to reciprocate beyond the call of duty. This can sometimes become a sticky situation and make your job more difficult to perform, especially since they are not your only patient. Don't panic, here are some suggestions:

- Be very clear that although you empathize with them and want the best for them, you also have the same ethic for all of your patients.

- Be very empathetic toward the patient's condition, but DO NOT encourage self-pity

- Have your Physical Therapist Assistant or PT Tech treat the patient as much as possible. This may help the patient become less "clingy" and dependent on you over time.

- Treat the patient while simultaneously treating another patient if possible. The patient may realize that they are not the only patient who needs your help, and feel the responsibility to "share" you with other patients.

- Empower the patient by rewarding any steps they take toward independence, and discouraging any steps they take toward dependence on you as the therapist.

- Explain to the patient that your role is as a mother bird who dedicates herself to raising her baby birds, but who knows that her only goal is to help them achieve the ability to leave the nest and fly on their own.

How do I deal with a situation where I am treating a patient who I have never seen, and who is usually treated by another therapist, says "the other therapist does it this way, why don't you do the same"? Are you sure you're doing this right?

Believe it or not, this is a very common complaint among patients, and a source of frustration among therapists. The patient only knows the treatment he/she has received in the past, and expects the same. However, they are not trained as you are, and are simply at a loss concerning proper intervention. Understandably, this is not a very comfortable situation for the patient. You don't want to seem as though you are incompetent, and you don't want the patient to think that they were receiving substandard care from the other therapist. So what do you do? Here are some suggestions:

- Explain to the patient that there are "more ways than one to get this job done".

- Explain that there is an art component in therapy and we each have a way we do things to achieve the same end result.

- Acknowledge the patients concern, and then explain why your treatment differs from the other therapist.

- Let the patient know that you treat the other therapist's patient's all the time. If the patient knows that his/her trusted physical therapist trust you, he/she will feel comfortable trusting you too, and will be more willing to accept your unique methods of treating them.

- Ease the patients mind by showing them common ground between yourself and the other therapist by explaining the diagnosis and prognosis of their condition to them. Then explain the various approaches to treatment including yours.

How do I deal with a situation where the aide/tech/assistant does things that I don't agree with, but was already trained to perform their job in that way before I was hired or came along?

This situation is almost always encountered by a therapist in a new position in one way or another, and immediately makes for a very uncomfortable and unwelcoming transition into the new position. Here are some suggestions by others who have gone through the same scenario.

- If it is not against company policy, against the well-being of the patient or others, try to do it the way it was initially being done. You might find that you agree that it is the best way to be done.

- If it has potential to harm yourself and others or if it is against company policy as a whole, inform your aide/tech/assistant why it should not be done, and tell them that you will need it to be done your way in the future.

- Remember that although you have had years of professional training, they may have years of practical experience. So be sure to first listen carefully to your aide/tech/assistant. There may be a moment where you can actually learn something from them.

- Avoid the "my way or the highway" speech. It only antagonizes the person you need to work with. Instead, explain to your "team mate" that both ways may work equally well, but you are at your best when doing it a certain way, just like the other therapists is at their best doing it their own way. Then ask them to try it your way.

- Try doing it once as suggested by your aide/tech. Then do it once in the method you suggest. Write down the pros and cons of both methods, and go over it with your aide/tech. Using this objective information, decide on which method is best, and stick to that method from then on.

- Tell your tech that you will be using your method for a while and if it doesn't work out by the end of the determined period of time (a week or a few months or so), you will try their suggested method. Chances are that your aide will eventually become accustomed to your method and actually allow it to work out better.

- Go to your supervisor and ask if there was a specific reason for the other method, and explain your suggested method. Ask them for their opinion, and then stick with that opinion.

How do I deal with a situation where I am asked by my supervisor or expected to do a certain thing, but believe it is illegal?

This almost never happens, and it is an extremely intimidating experience for a new physical therapist who only recently passed his/her PT board exam. You certainly do not want to compromise your principals and professional ethics. And you most certainly don't want to risk losing that physical therapy license that you recently obtained, framed and hung on the wall. At the same time, you don't want to do the wrong thing by overreacting to the situation, causing unnecessary friction at your job and maybe even lose your job. For this reason, it is important to know that other physical therapists have found themselves in this situation, and have emerged without a scratch because they implemented successful strategies that they created. They want to offer you their strategies because it is comforting and empowering to know what to do if the situation arises. The following are suggestions:

- Just say NO!!!

- You don't want to embarrass yourself by making something out of nothing. So, the first thing you should do if you're not sure is research the subject to determine if it is indeed illegal. Remember, you could be wrong or simply be misinformed.

- Ask other physical therapists (more than one) to give you their opinion about what you should do. It may be a good idea to ask a therapist who not associated with your job, though.

- Remember that it's YOUR license to practice physical therapy that is on the line. You did not go through all of those years of school only to have your license revoked or go to jail.

- Tell your supervisor that you are not comfortable with the task, and why. Then ask them to allow time for you to research it before you decide on what you should do. Most supervisors have many years of experience, and know legal versus illegal things relevant to physical therapy. They also know that you are a new therapist who may not be well versed in the law. They will probably respect your decision, and grant you the time to research. If after research, you find that it is indeed illegal, copy the data and show it to your supervisor personally to back up your decision to refuse. If you are wrong, apologize and move forward. Either way, you can't lose because a good supervisor will probably gain respect for you in the end.

Tips on how to get a nervous patient to relax muscle tone so that manual therapy can be performed?

Your patient injured their upper trapezius musculature and has upper trapezius spasm and severe tightness that limits their ability to lower their shoulder. You decide to utilize soft tissue mobilization/functional massage as part of your treatment plan, but your patient is so nervous and anxious that they won't allow you to touch them without jumping and squirming away from your touch. Happens all the time, and there are many time-proven methods to alleviate this problem, and most of these methods are as simple as the following.

- Dim the lights lighten the atmosphere.

- If the diagnosis is a soft tissue-related injury, apply electrical stimulation and moist heat to the treatment area first, then proceed from there.

"Before you begin, explain exactly what you will be doing, and why. This helps ease the patient's apprehension". Jordan Alfrey, DPT. Lewiston, ID.

- Tell funny jokes to break the ice

- Make sure music is playing in the background.

- Let them know that although it may be uncomfortable at first, it will not hurt.

- I instruct the patient to let me know JUST BEFORE it gets uncomfortable, and I will make adjustments.

- Start out extremely light in order to belay their apprehension of pain

- Divert their attention by discussing their children, how they got injured, years of marriage, weather, etc.

- Explain that a relaxed body may benefit more, thus speeding their recovery time.

Tips on avoiding an "awkward discharge" so pt won't think you are just trying to get rid of them?

You have been treating your patient for weeks now, and consequently, their condition has resolved. But now you have to tell the patient that you will no longer be seeing him/her. It's almost like breaking up with someone you have been dating for a short period, it has a very high potential for massive awkwardness. But unlike breaking up with a girlfriend/boyfriend, there are actually steps to take that can significantly reduce or completely remove all traces of awkwardness. Take it from physical therapists that have done this thousands of times, these methods work. So, let's see what they are.

- It starts at initial evaluation. You MUST make sure that the two of you agree on the goals you want to accomplish during PT. Make them understand that the reason they are in therapy is to accomplish their goals. If you are discharging them because they have reached all of their goals, let the pt know that you are happy they have reached their goals, and that PT is no longer needed. If you are discharging the patient because they have failed to reach their goals, and it is your professional opinion that they do not have the potential to reach them, make sure you carefully inform them of this during a one-on-one re-evaluation session. If you are discharging them because of insurance restrictions, non-compliance, change in health status, or any other reason, you should inform them of the exact reason during a one-on-one session. In this way, the patient is assured that you don't just want to get rid of them, and is comfortable with the knowledge that you are competently performing your job.

- Be sure to give them something to take home with them that will continue to help them such as written instructions, home exercise program, list of local exercise or water aerobics facilities, or walking cane.

- Make sure they know that you will still just be a phone call away if they have any questions or concerns about their condition.

- If you are contemplating discharge within the next few sessions, let the patient know a few sessions prior to the actual

164

day of discharge so that they will be expecting it and won't be taken by surprise.

- Go out to the waiting room and say goodbye to the patient's family or friends.

- Let them know that you will be contacting their referring doctor either by phone, mail, or fax to inform them of their status.

- In addition to physically preparing the patient for discharge, help the patient mentally and physically prepare themselves for discharge by discussing the probability of discharge well in advance of the actual date of discharge. In this way, there will be no surprises, and things should go very smoothly.

- To help ease the patients tension during this transition phase, I always ask the patient in a joking way "what are you going to do with all the time you are going to have on your hands after today since you won't have to come to therapy anymore?" They almost always joke back saying something to the effect of "now that I'm free from this place, I can finally do this or that", we laugh and shake hands, and that's that. Done deal.

Tips on how to tell if a person is faking their injuries or problems?

Unfortunately, there are some who seek physical therapy for reasons other than what they tell us. The two most common reasons people fake injuries is for emotional sympathy and for financial gain. I have heard this referred to as Symptom Magnification Syndrome Type 1 and Type 2. Type one is for emotional support (such as after a loved one dies or to relieve emotional stress) while type two is for financial gain (such as suing an auto insurance company for injuries purportedly sustained during a motor vehicle accident). It is important to remember be very careful when using the phrase "faking" because in my experience, most people who fake injuries probably do, in fact, have an injury. However, it may not be as bad as they would like you to believe. So one must treat the condition based on your objective findings, while keeping in mind that subjective information may be biased but not totally bogus.

- Compare actual objectively obtained measurement with subjective reports, if they don't match, the person may be exaggerating.

- Remember to write down all of the facts the patient reports, and follow-up with the same questions a week or so later. If there is a change in the story, the patient could have SMS Type 1 or type 2.

- Very casually ask the family members or friends of the patient a few of the same questions while they are in the same room or at a later time during treatment. Don't ask them outside of the presence of the patient because they will probably tell the patient that you inquired about the facts, and the patient may perceive that as distrust.

- Don't ask "leading" questions which may steer the patient's answers one way or another. For example, instead of saying "does this hurt?" say "how does this feel?" or "what happens when I do this?". A person who is not malingering will simply answer by stating how it feels to them, while a person who is malingering usually tends to report pain with everything tested. This technique works especially well with special tests for radiculopathy because patients may be unaware of dermatome and myotome distribution.

- Pay close attention to patient's posture, guarding, etc. before, during, and immediately after therapy sessions. Some patients who are malingering often forget to keep up the appearance of being in pain or dysfunctional.

- Frequently ask the patient to remind you of the circumstances which caused the injury. Some malingering patients may forget the original story, and create a partially different story. If the story changes frequently for no apparent reason, you can suspect malingering or symptom magnification.

166

How do I deal with a boss who makes me do things that I believe I shouldn't or feel uncomfortable doing them.

Don't worry, this happens all the time, and it is not necessarily a bad thing. Remember that honesty, in this case, is always the best policy. If you are dishonest, it will eventually be discovered, and you will then lose valuable credibility and your boss will lose confidence in your competence.

- If your reason for discomfort is because you honestly believe it should not be done for ethical or legal reasons, etc., communicate your feelings with your boss in a private place, and explain why you feel this way (refer to answer #90).

- If you don't feel comfortable doing the requested thing because you feel you are not experienced enough yet, ask your boss for alternatives such as doing it with another veteran therapist for the first time, and then alone after you become comfortable with it.

- If you are uncomfortable because you simply don't know how to do it, don't be afraid to tell the truth. Your boss will usually understand that you are a new therapist, and may still have some learning to do. They will probably be happy to invest their time and resources in teaching you how to do it because it is ultimately in their own best interests. It is also in your own best interest.

- If you have not been asked yet, but you know that you will be asked soon, be proactive. Look it up, and review it before you are asked to do it. If you still feel uncomfortable, be sure to let your supervisor know that you don't have a lot of experience with it, but do understand it very well (because you read up on it first). This should take the pressure of expectation off of your shoulders and alleviate some of the nervousness.

- If you are too nervous to do it, simply tell your boss that this is your first time doing it, and your too nervous. Tell your them that you would like to see him/her do it first so that you can be sure that your doing it correctly. Then carefully imitate the way they do it. Later, be sure to practice independently again until you are very comfortable with it.

The most important things to have memorized in hospital setting:

As a physical therapist who works in a hospital setting, there are certain things that if memorized, can actually help make you a better physical therapist.

- It goes without saying, but normal heart rate, normal blood pressure, normal respiratory rate, CPR

- How to pause and shut off the alarm on the Automatic IV fluid machine.

- Professional in charge of the patient's immediate care (nurse in charge, Pt's doctor, nurse's aide, etc.).

- As many JACHO safety rules as possible .

- All safety codes (Blue, Green, Red, etc.), and the correct corresponding procedure

- Location of MSD

- Code procedure for medical emergency

- Signs of medical emergency (near syncope while gait training, orthostatic hypotension, seizure, etc.)

- Standard procedure for medical emergency concerning the patient under your care

- How to contact your patient's nurse via the appropriate communications devices (pagers, nurse call button, nurse cell phones, etc.) the hospital utilizes.

The most important things to have memorized in an outpatient setting:

Just like in the hospital setting, there are certain things that physical therapists should have memorized well in order to be a great outpatient physical therapist. According to physical therapists who have worked in outpatient setting for many years, these are the things you should memorize.

- At least two special tests for everybody joint

- Deep tendon reflex scale

- Normal ROM for all joints

- Special joint mobilization techniques for all joints

- CPR

- Hip Replacement post-surgical precautions

- General ACL post-op rehab protocol

- General shoulder labrum post-op rehab protocol

- Vendor for ordering DME such as orthopedic braces, assistive devices such as canes, etc.

The most important things to have memorized in a neurological Physical Therapy setting:

The neurological physical therapy setting is a very unique PT setting, and as such, it is very useful and wise to memorize certain specific items. According to veteran neuro PTs, memorizing the following items will greatly help improve your practice in this setting.

- Deep tendon reflex scale

- Myotome screen tests for all spinal levels

- Locations to screen/test all dermatomes.

- Procedures for testing all cranial nerves

- Tests for mental status changes

- Dix-Hallpike Maneuver

- Rhomberg Test

- How to test for Nystagmus

- Spasticity scale

- Heel-Shin Test

- Finger-to-nose test

- Rapid Alternating Movement Test

- Overshoot Test

- Get up and Go test

- The Spastic Paraplegia Rating Scale (SPRS)

- American Spinal Injury Association (ASIA) score/scale

The most important things to have memorized in a subacute rehab setting such as a nursing home:

Ahh yes, the subacute rehab facility. Unique in its own way, and as with all other settings, memorizing certain things will help improve your practice as a physical therapist. So, consider remembering the following if you work in the subacute rehab setting.

- Efficient transfer techniques

- Normal heart rate

- Normal Blood pressure

- Normal respiratory rate

- Fall prevention techniques and advice

- CPR

- Sternal precautions

- Hip precautions

- Emergency code procedures

The most important things to remember in a sports therapy setting:

The sports physical therapy setting is similar to the outpatient physical therapy setting, but usually requires higher level of everything because, although the patients are injured, their current and expected level of physical activity is still higher than the typical patient in a non-sport outpatient setting. This being said, there are things relative to this setting that a physical therapist should have memorized that will help him/her be a better PT. with this in mind, I submit the following to you.

- Taping techniques

- ACSM guidelines strength, endurance, and stretching

- Host of creative, advanced, high level, and sport-specific exercises

- CPR

- Names of most common sport related injuries

- Standard treatment interventions for most common sport related injuries

- All rules of the specific game or sport activity, and how to play/participate

- How to operate sport braces/sport equipment, etc.

- Standard protocol for emergency injury situation

The most important things to remember in a home care setting:

Home care setting does not require anywhere near as much memorization as all of the other PT settings. However, there are still things that, if memorized, can help you be a better physical therapist in the home care setting. The following is a list of those things.

- Normal Blood pressure

- Normal Heart rate

- CPR

- Make sure patient signs documentation

- Make sure there is a designated spacious area for exercise.

- Try to avoid accepting anything to eat or drink from the patient, especially home-made food

- Always wash hands and use instant hand sanitizer before you leave the patient's home

- Be creative and fun with the exercise so the patient will look forward to your next visit.

- Familiarize yourself with and remember the names of the patient's family and other caretakers

- If the television is on, turn it off. It will distract the patient and make you appear distracted also.

- Have the patient's family's telephone numbers readily accessible in case of emergency.

- Even though your already scheduled to be there at a certain time, call the pt before you come.

- Always coordinate your intervention with the visiting nurse, speech, or OT.

- Make sure all documentation is done before you leave the home.

- Take vital signs at first sign of a problem

- Don't forget the blood pressure cuff and stethoscope

- Don't allow family or other persons in the house distract you or the patient

- Make the patient understand that the time your there should be strictly dedicated to therapy.

- If you feel unsafe in the patient's home, inform your supervisor immediately.

- Help the pt, but resist the urge to do their chores (taking out trash, dishes, cleaning house, etc.).

What are some suggested ways to document the fact that my patient is making steady progress?

Documenting patient progress on a daily level is essential to the process of rehabilitation. The problem is that actually putting it in words can be so tediously repetitive that it makes you want to jump off a cliff. Don't worry, years of documenting patient's progress as veteran physical therapists has resulted in a Patient progress documentation "cheat sheet" for you. Enjoy.

- "Pt's gait appeared less antalgic and safer today with improved balance control".

- "Pt c/o less discomfort during exercise today"

- "Pt was able to remove his coat with only minimal assistance today".

- "Pt states that he was able to perform the exercises in the home program with less difficulty".

- "Pt was able to perform the (specific exercise) with much less difficulty today".

- "Pt is showing improved cervical posture today as seen with less cervical flexion".

- "Pt no longer needs a cane for ambulation"

- "Pt states that he was able to drive for the first time since the injury today".

- "Pt was able to use a fork to eat with only minimal difficulty for the first time today".

- "Pt was able to tie shoes for the first time since surgery today".

- "Pt showing improved trunk posture today, as seen with less trunk flexion during ambulation".

- "Pt appeared less apprehensive about stair/gait training today".

- "Pt was able to carry his suitcase in to work today with only minimal difficulty yesterday".

- "Pt was able to demonstrate independence with initial level HEP today".

- "Pt was able to partial squat with only mild/moderate difficulty to pick up his keys today".

- "Pt was able to wear regular gym shoes without significant foot pain for the first time today".

- "Pt is now requiring less assistance with donning her coat".

- "Pt states that she was able to use injured arm to brush hair for the first time today".

- "Pt was able to bend forward with much less difficulty in order to tie shoes today".

- "Pt is now able to sit in a single position for longer without shifting weight due to discomfort".

- "Pt states that she was able to walk up 5 stairs at home without the assistance of her son".

- "Pt can now ascend stairs using reciprocal gait, but still requires railings or physical assistance".

- "Pt able to hold plate of food using involved hand with only minimal assistance from opposite hand".

- "Pt states, although still difficult, he is able to reach further when washing his back in shower".

- "Pt states that he was able to sit long enough to watch a movie for the first time since surgery".

- "Pt now able to fit involved foot into show with less difficulty".

- "Pt states that she was able to use a spoon to eat yesterday for the first time since the stroke".

- "Pt states that he was able to rotate neck enough to look behind him when attempting to park his car".

- "Pt is now able to use involved hand to button shirt with much less difficulty".

- "Pt now only needs one rest break during gait training".

- "Pt now requires cane less, as he frequently forgets to bring it with him when leaving the home".

- "Pt now using involved hand when signing his name, and more legibly".

- "Pt transitioning sit to stand with less effort, and is less dependent on the walker to do so".

- "Pt now appears to be bearing more weight into the involved ankle with ambulation".

- "Pt now transitioning supine to sit without assistance from therapist, and with less effort".

Special thanks to the following Physical Therapists for contributing the benefits of their many years of experience in the field of physical therapy to the content of this book.

Cynthia Bell, PT, DPT. Valdosta GA

Steven D. Goostree, PT, DPT, OCS, FAAOMPT. Chicago Il

Jaisie Stevens, PT, DPT. Washington DC

Brian Mabrey, MSPT. Brooklyn, NY

David Bullock, MPT. Silver Spring, MD

Darryl Elliott, PT. Milton, MA

Darryl Elliott, PT, DPT, OCS. Orange CA

Darlene Orangias, PT, DPT. Louisvile, KY

Cynthia Dvorsky, MPT. Clinton, CT

Alan J. Howell, PT, SCS, ATC. Cincinnati, OH

Gregory Hullstrung, Gregory Hullstrung. Mohegan Lake, NY

Scott Roberts, PT, MPT, MS, COMT, CMTPT, MCMT, CMT. Richmond, VA

Brett Rice, MPT, FAAOMPT. New Market MD

Irene Drizi, PT. Athens, Greece

Natalie Maharaj, MPT. Annandale, VA

Kira Davis, PT Silver Spring, MD

Daniel Curtis, PT, DPT, MTC. Orlando, FL

Simina Bono, BHSc., PT, DPT, OCS, Troy, MI

Rhonda White, MSPT. Chicago, IL

Eric Mabbagu, PT, DPT. Orlando, FL

Felipe R. Singco, Jr. PT, Antipolo City, Philippines

Juan Di Leo Razuk, PT, CMP, Cert. MDT, DPT, CMPT. Valparaiso, IN

Kim Braun, PT, DPT. Beaverton, OR

Kim Braun, PT, MA, DPT. Ridgewood, NY

Theresa A. Schmidt, PT,DPT,MS,OCS,LMT,CEAS,CHY. Northport, NY

Jordan Alfrey, DPT. Lewiston, ID

Ray Berardinelli, MPT. Claysburg, PA

Eric Wanner, PT, DPT, OCS. West Palm Beach, FL

West Palm Beach, DPT. Waterford, MI

Ian Manning, MSPT. North Kingstown, RI

Susan McNamara, PT, MMSc. South Portland, ME

Giselle Defreitas, MPT. Washington, DC

Brenda Rapuano, PT. Wallingford, CT

Adil Irani, MPT. Hagerstown, MD

Venise Mule-Glass, PT,DPT,OCS,CSCS. Commack, NY

Alex Pandya, MPT. Rochester, MI

Yvonne Tracie, PT, Waldorf, MD

Riggolette Leeper, MPT. Decatur, GA

Monique A. Myers, PT, DPT. Wilmington DE

Donald Phillips, PTA. Belleville, MI

Danladi Whitten, MPT. Washington, DC

Jay Neal, PT. BelAir, MD

Van Watts, MPT. Greenbelt, MD

If you would like to be listed as a contributing physical therapist in the next edition of Practical Solutions for the New Physical Therapist, go to **https://www.surveymonkey.com/r/theptsurvey**, and fill out the questionaire.